THE CANNABIS
PRESCRIPTION

How to Use MEDICAL MARIJUANA to Reduce
or Replace Pharmaceutical Medications

THE **CANNABIS**
PRESCRIPTION

How to Use MEDICAL MARIJUANA to Reduce or Replace Pharmaceutical Medications

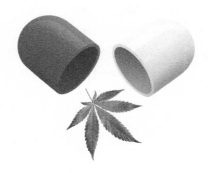

Colleen Higgins, R.Ph.

DISCLAIMER

Everything contained in this book, written content, images and graphics are to be used for informational purposes only. The content is not meant to diagnose or substitute for medical advice from a licensed healthcare provider. Please do not disregard advice provided by your doctor or delay in recommended treatment to follow advice given in this book. Seek medical attention immediately if wounded, in pain, or injuries or disease worsen after using cannabis. All names and identifying information have been changed to protect patient privacy.

Neither the author nor publisher shall be held liable or responsible in any capacity for injury, loss, or damage sustained from the use of this book. If injured, sick, wounded, or mentally confused, immediately seek medical attention at your nearest emergency room.

MED 00400
HEA 053000
REF 030000

Paperback ISBN 978-1-7340034-4-4
E-book ISBN 978-1-7340034-0-6
LCCN: 2019913283
Published by Sway Innovations
URL: SwayInnovations.com

Cover and interior design by David Provolo

For all the patients who struggle with lost hope

and

my beautiful daughter, Grace

Table of Contents

SECTION 1
The Cannabis Plant

Chapter 1

Man's Relationship with Hemp

The Criminalization of Cannabis

1937: Cannabis Was Made Illegal—The First Time

Pharmaceuticals Are Big, Big, Big Bu$ine$$

How the Opioid Epidemic Came to Life

Big Pharma's Cannabis: Epidiolex: Plant-Based,
   FDA-Approved CBD

Chapter 2

The Endocannabinoid Receptor System (ERS) and
   Its Impact on Health
      Endocannabinoid System Responses in the Human Body

Trichomes

Decarboxylation of Cannabinoids: Activate!

Cannabinoids Available in Dispensaries

Cannabinoid Applications (THC, CBD, CBN, and THCA)

The Prescription THC Pill: Why Not Just Get That?

The Entourage Effect

The Role of Terpenes

Indica, Hybrid, and Sativa Strains

Hemp Oil versus Hemp Extract versus Phytocannabinoid-Rich
   Hemp Oil (PCR)

Conduction versus Convection Vaporizers
How to Use a Vaporizer
Portable versus Tabletop Vaporizers
Definition of "Cannabis Oil"
Concentrates/Wax/Shatter/Budder/Live Resin/Rosin/Dabs/Sauce
Pre-Filled Vapor Pens (No Additional Battery Required)
Oil Vapor Cartridges (Additional Battery Required)
    CO_2 Oil Cartridges
    Distillate Oil Cartridges
    Live Resin Oil Cartridges
Diluents Used in Oil Cartridges: Know What's In Your Cartridge
Vapor Cartridge Hardware Styles
Pre-Filled Cartridges versus Fill-It-Yourself Cartridges
Everything You Need to Know About Batteries for Cartridges
Quick Tips to Get the Most Out of Your Battery

Chapter 5

Sublingual Products Available in Dispensaries
    Oils
    Tinctures
    Solutions
How to Calculate Your Dose Using a Liquid Product
    Elixirs
    Sprays
    Sublingual Slips or Films

Chapter 6

Why Edibles Produce Stronger Psychotropic Effects Than Inhalation
    or Sublingual Dosing
The Effects of Combining Alcohol and THC Edibles
Translating Cannabis Tincture as an Edible
CBD and THC "Water Soluble" Nano-emulsions and Micro-emulsions
Homemade Edibles
How To Calculate Milligrams (mg) of THC in Cannabis Flower

Topical Products for Treating Radiation Burns
CBD and THC Use in Killing Cancer Cells (RSO)
How CBD May Help Prevent Chemotherapy-Induced Organ Damage

CBD for REM Behavioral Disturbances
Cannabis for "Freeze"
Cannabis for Pain
Cannabis for Emotional Issues

The Endocannabinoid System's Role in Epilepsy
Pharmaceutical Treatments for Epilepsy: Anti-Epileptic Drugs (AEDs)
AED Drug Interactions with Cannabis
CBD Treatments for Seizure Disorders
Dispensary Cannabis Oil versus Pharmaceutical Products
THC Use in Epilepsy and Treatment of Active Seizure
THCA Treatment for Seizure Disorders
Beginning CBD Therapy
How to Determine Optimal Daily Dosage of CBD

Pharmaceutical Treatments for Anxiety and Depression
    Problems with Benzodiazepines or "Benzos"
Cannabis Treatments for Anxiety and Depression
    Best Cannabis for Treating Anxiety
    A Layered Approach to Treating Anxiety
    Best Cannabis for Depression
        Start with CBD
        Adding THC

Pharmaceutical Treatments for Gastrointestinal Disorders
Cannabis Treatments for Gastrointestinal Disorders
    Inflammation and Spasms
    Nausea and Vomiting
    Anal Fissures

Timing Inhaled Doses

Breathe in slowly 1 puff (2-3 seconds in duration) maximum. Do not keep inhaling or you risk over consumption.

You will feel the effects within 1-15 minutes.

If the dose is too low, re-medicate with 1-2 puffs after 20 to 30 minutes.

Effects from inhalation last from 1-3 hours. Medicate as needed.

Timing Sublingual Doses

Apply under the tongue or between cheek and gum. Do not eat or drink for 10-15 minutes after dose.

You will notice the effect within 5-30 minutes.

If the dose is too low, re-medicate after 3 hours.

The effects of sublingual products can last 3-4 hours.

If accidentally swallowed, sublinguals work like edibles, so be sure to place under the tongue or between the cheek and gum.

Timing Edible Doses

Take with a small amount of food but not on a full stomach, or the effect will be delayed.

Liquid products will work slightly faster than foods.

Onset is between 45 minutes and 2 hours.

Do not re-dose for 6 hours, especially if this is your first time taking an edible.

Edibles last from 4-12 hours depending on the patient. Most patients experience the effects of edibles for 4-6 hours.

Higher and excessive dosages can last longer than lower dosages, so it is important to find your most comfortable and effective dose.

How to Micro-Dose

	Inhalation	Sublingual	Edible
Starting Dose	Take one (2-4 second) puff.	Take 1mg of CBD and THC.	Take 1mg of CBD and THC.
Frequency	every 6 hours	every 8 hours	every 8-12 hours
Increasing Dose	Increase number of puffs or frequency until effective.	Increase by 1mg of both THC and CBD every 5 to 7 days.	Increase by 1mg of both THC and CBD every 5 to 7 days.

How to Calculate Your Dose Using a Liquid Product

Divide total (mg) in bottle by the total (ml) in bottle = mg in 1 ml.

This is the milligrams in 1ml of your tincture. If a 1ml dose is too high, then calculate the following:

0.5ml = mg in ml divided by 2

0.25ml = mg in ml divided by 4

How to Calculate Milligrams (mg) of THC or CBD in Cannabis Flower

(1000 x %THC from label) x grams of flower = amount of THC in your flower

Example: 14 grams of 18% THC flower is
1000 x 0.18=180mg THC x 14grams

This equals 2520 milligrams of THC total

Introduction

"Natural forces within us are the true healers of disease."
Hippocrates[1]

As a patient in today's healthcare system, have you tried pill after pill after pill in an attempt to relieve symptoms only to find that you feel worse? Does it seem like the only option you have when you visit your doctor is another expensive pill, and that's no longer an option for you?

Well, my friend, the tide has turned.

Through grassroots efforts only and in spite of government interference, medical cannabis use has increased exponentially over the last two decades as the fear and propaganda of the 1930s is replaced by overwhelming scientific data that supports claims regarding the safety and efficacy of cannabis as a valuable medical asset.

No longer is the only choice for medicine isolated to Big Pharma products.

Cannabis research, beginning with the discovery of the Endocannabinoid Receptor System (ERS), is emerging as a new area of scientific study in the treatment of pain, chemotherapy side effects, glaucoma, anxiety, depression, and much more—all the while being safer, more effective, and often less expensive when compared to what is sold in pharmacies today.

As a pharmacist, I have dispensed and compounded drugs for almost thirty years. In that time, I discovered that a significant portion of patients being treated in our healthcare system are often left disappointed, suffering, and underwhelmed by drug options available in insurance sanctioned healthcare.

If you go to a surgeon, they will want to cut. If you go to your doctor, you expect to get a Big Pharma prescription. Somehow, someway America has been engulfed in prescription drugs, which, while highly profitable for the pharmaceutical industry, are not proving to be the most beneficial choice for patients in the long run.

A Pew analysis showed that between 2012 and 2016, net spending on drugs sold in pharmacies rose from $250.7 billion to $341 billion.[2] That's more than the GDP of most countries on Earth. Business is booming! According to the Mayo Clinic and Olmsted Medical Center, more than 70% of Americans are on at least one prescription drug while more than 50% take at least two medications.[3] Being on a prescription pill is the norm when you live in America.

The problem is, living on all these pharmaceutical drugs does not necessarily equate to a longer and healthier life. The Central Intelligence Agency website lists the United States life expectancy in 2017 as #43 in the world, well below countries like Spain (#22), Italy (#15), and Ireland (#33).[4]

We spend more on drugs and healthcare than any other country in the world, yet we are #43 for life expectancy? Something is not adding up.

I wrote *The Cannabis Prescription* after helping thousands of patients find relief through the proper use of medical cannabis after trying every pill on the market with little to no success. Emerging science can be confusing and patients dealing with debilitating conditions need guidance when learning how to use cannabis properly, specifically THC and CBD, the two cannabinoids found in highest concentrations in the plant. Walking into a cannabis dispensary is intimidating and overwhelming for most people, which is why many patients choose to stick it out with what's dispensed in pharmacies. I designed this book to educate patients who have limited exposure to cannabis about subjects including:

- the history of cannabis in the United States, specifically how the criminalization of cannabis was never actually based in science (Hint: Follow the money.);

- cannabis plant strains (indica, hybrid, and sativa) and why it's important to know the difference (unless you want to sleep all day);
- the Endocannabinoid Receptor System (ERS) and how these receptors influence our mood, eyesight, fear response, cardiac function, diabetes development, pain response, fertility, and much more;
- the cannabinoids contained within the cannabis plant, specifically CBD (cannabidiol), THC (Δ-9-tetrahydrocannabinol), THCA (tetrahydrocannabinolic acid), and a relatively unknown molecule CBN (cannabinol), which are found in products sold in most cannabis dispensaries across the country;
- how to effectively use the main ingredient of industrial hemp, CBD (cannabidiol), which was legalized in December of 2018, and clear up the confusion about the differences between hemp oil, hemp extract, and PCR (Phyto-Cannabinoid Rich Hemp Oil);
- why choose an inhaled product versus an edible, along with specific directions on how to safely, comfortably, and effectively administer cannabis by inhalation, sublingual dose, and when taking an edible;
- how to adjust your dose when it is not working or feels too strong;
- and how to alleviate the most common symptoms of diseases for which cannabis has been shown to be effective, such as Parkinson's disease, treatment of chronic pain, relief from chemotherapy side effects, migraine treatment and prevention, gastrointestinal issues, anxiety, sleep, and more.

Currently, cannabis is considered a last option in healthcare and *The Cannabis Prescription* reveals how it needs to be recognized as a potential first choice.

If you have been suffering from ineffective therapeutic options when treating a healthcare concern, whatever it may be, there is a real possibility that cannabis can offer some positive relief. Unlike pharmaceuticals, it is a natural fit for our body's own Endocannabinoid Receptor System

(ERS). Often the best answer for patients when treating a malady is to have as many options available to them as possible. I refer to it as more tools in the toolbox. There is never a "one size fits all" answer for anything in life, especially when it comes to our medicine.

Knowledge is power, and this book offers everything you need to know when learning to navigate a cannabis dispensary and begin using cannabis to heal your body. Once you learn how to get the most out of the cannabis plant, you can begin to take control of how you medicate at a time when everything can feel very much out of control.

We begin our journey by looking back to a time when cannabis was celebrated as a safe, effective medicine sold in pharmacies across America until racist beliefs and inflammatory propaganda stripped away its value and replaced it with fear and criminalization. The next chapter is heavy on history, so if you wish to dive straight into how to use cannabis as medicine, skip to chapter 2.

SECTION 1

The Cannabis Plant

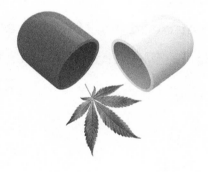

Cannabis first entered the U.S. Pharmacopoeia in 1850 (3rd edition). It was removed in 1942 as a result of the 1937 Marihuana Tax Act drafted by Harry Anslinger.

CHAPTER 1

Cannabis History and Fighting for a Future

*"Laws and institutions must go hand in hand with the progress
of the human mind, as that becomes more developed, more enlightened,
as new discoveries are made, more truths discovered and manners
and opinions change, with the change of circumstance, institutions
must advance also to keep pace with the times."*
Thomas Jefferson[1]

Marijuana. Weed. Pot. Reefer. Grass. Ganja. Maryjane. Giggle smoke. The devil's lettuce. Time.com reports that people use over *1,200* different slang terms for a plant that should simply be called cannabis.[2] In addition to its many names, just as many myths surround the plant. Cannabis, along with the cultivated hop (used in beer), is part of the botanical family of Cannabaceae, and is thought to have originated in Asia over 5,000 years ago. Its multiple uses in medicine and beyond steadily made its way across the globe. A recent report told of the discovery of an entombed man from 2500 BC who was buried in China with thirteen cannabis plants shrouded across his body, revealing the depths to which this plant has been celebrated since a time when medicine was only provided from the earth.

Man's Relationship with Hemp

Hemp is a distinct species of the *Cannabis sativa* plant that historically has been grown for industrial use due to its strong fibers and multiple functions. There are hundreds of strains of cannabis; hemp contains less than 0.3 % of the psychoactive cannabinoid THC (Δ-9-tetrahydrocannabinol) and higher concentrations of the non-psychoactive component CBD (cannabidiol). Both hemp and marijuana fall under the classification of cannabis, with other strains containing higher concentrations of THC (at the time around 3-4%).

Cannabis played a major role in the development of North America, including both Canada and the US. In the American colonies, cannabis was a renewable source used for textiles, paper, rope, and medicine. George Washington said, "I am very glad to hear that the Gardener has saved so much of the St. foin seed, and that of the India Hemp. Make the most you can of both....The Hemp may be sown anywhere."[3]

So, what changed? Why did hemp go from a valuable resource to a "dangerous substance" that needed to be removed from society just recently? For centuries across the globe, cannabis has been celebrated and utilized. Yet in just the last eighty years it has been devalued and criminalized by those in power. Why this sudden shift in perspective? What made the government turn against a plant with so many established benefits? Well, in a capitalistic culture such as ours, all we need to do is follow the money to see who profits when access to cannabis is removed from society.

The Criminalization of Cannabis

Beginning in the eighteenth century, cotton production overtook hemp production because of the difficulty in harvesting the tough, durable fibers of the hemp plant. The patenting of Eli Whitney's cotton gin in 1794 tipped the scales toward cotton production, but in 1917 American George W. Schlichten patented a new machine for separating the hemp fiber from the internal woody core or "hurds", thus reducing the labor costs one hundred times and increasing the fiber yield by sixty times.[4]

Interestingly, Mr. Schlichten's new machine never seemed to catch on. Unfortunately for him, his invention coincided with the condemning government attitude toward cannabis in response to increased immigration from Mexico at the beginning of the twentieth century. The paranoia surrounding cannabis was evident just two years after his invention when in 1919 Texas outlawed cannabis, and it has been widely reported a senator on the floor of the Senate said: "all Mexicans are crazy, and this stuff (marijuana) is what makes them crazy." The criminalization of cannabis had begun, and it was firmly built on the grounds of racism and fear, never based in science.

As well as being tied to what was considered the underclass, the hundreds of products derived from hemp such as rope, paper, textiles, and bird feed were in direct competition with the interests of large, powerful corporate families like the Duponts with their synthetic fibers (nylon) and the Hearst empire, which contained massive timberlands and mills to produce paper and newspaper. I have found articles that show how hemp can be used to produce up to twenty thousand different products. A plastic developed by Ford chemists for Henry Ford's first Model-T automobile used hemp (and other materials) that, when combined, created a product with an impact strength ten times greater than steel.[5]

But many in power found the diversity of hemp a threat to their livelihood. Hemp products which could be easily and inexpensively produced made cannabis a big headache for companies as politically powerful as Dupont and Hearst, and they, along with emerging pharmaceutical companies, aimed to eliminate cannabis from society.

Enter Harry Anslinger, the first man appointed to head the Federal Narcotics Bureau (FNB, a precursor to the DEA) in 1930. The FNB was formed to uphold the prohibition on alcohol that had begun in 1920. Anslinger aligned himself with Washington insiders, including the Dupont and Hearst families, as well as the burgeoning pharmaceutical industry. His policies of prohibition, racism, hate, and zeal for law and order were the building blocks of modern drug policy and inspired the failed Reagan "War on Drugs" fifty years later.

Once alcohol prohibition ended in 1933, Anslinger needed to create a new threat in order to retain funds for his hard-line agency. Since there were few users of cocaine and heroin at the time, he set his sights on cannabis and its use within the minority communities. With little evidence to back up his claims, he used his office to promote an association between marijuana and violence. He tried to sell the idea that if a person used cannabis, they were more likely to be a crazed and violent criminal.

Initially, his "reefer madness" approach was effective. Fear, as anyone can attest, is an extremely effective motivator. In 1936, the movie *Reefer Madness* was created as a propaganda piece that promoted the message that cannabis made people crazy.[6] But, when the mayor of New York, Fiorello LaGuardia, commissioned a group of doctors to research Anslinger's claims, they concluded that everything Anslinger spewed was unequivocally false. "The LaGuardia Report" of 1944 showed no link between violent crime and the use of cannabis.[7]

Never one to give in to truth, Anslinger simply switched his dialogue from one of crazed, violent criminals to cannabis being equivalent to "dope" or heroin, an unsubstantiated overreach designed to keep people scared from a benign plant. In a radio address, he said young people were "slaves to this narcotic, continuing addiction until they deteriorate mentally, become insane, turn to violent crime and murder."[8] The aggressive, inflammatory, and racist Anslinger mentality influenced drug policy through the end of the twenty-first century with policies based on criminalization and incarceration of drug users. We can see his influence woven throughout the Reagan drug policies of the 1980s and beyond.

1937: Cannabis Was Made Illegal—The First Time

Anslinger's first maneuver to make cannabis an illegal substance came when he drafted the Marihuana Tax Act of 1937. With this act, people were not permitted to sell or use cannabis without exposing themselves to arrest, thus removing its legal use throughout the country. The Marihuana Tax Act was deemed unconstitutional in 1969 when Harvard educated psychologist Timothy Leery was arrested for possession of cannabis at the Mexican border and argued that the Act itself was a violation of the Fifth Amendment by requiring self-incrimination.[9]

After the Marihuana Tax Act was overturned in 1969, President Nixon responded with the Controlled Substances Act of 1970. Against the recommendation of the American Medical Association, Nixon classified cannabis as a Federal Schedule 1 drug. For him, drugs were "public enemy number one" and removal from society was paramount. Schedule 1 drugs are "drugs, substances, or chemicals [that] are defined by the federal government as drugs with no currently accepted medical use and a high potential for abuse. Schedule 1 drugs are the most dangerous drugs of all the drug schedules with potentially severe psychological or physical dependence."[10] By classifying cannabis as a Schedule 1 substance, Nixon essentially removed all of its potential benefits, present, and future, from society. A Schedule 1 substance cannot be prescribed. More importantly, research cannot be conducted to discover a Schedule 1 drug's untapped medical value. It looked as if this might be the final blow to the legality of cannabis.

To support his claims that cannabis is a dangerous substance with no medical value, Nixon, in 1971, had Congress commission a group of anti-drug researchers to conduct an extensive examination into the scientific documentation already available. Unfortunately for Nixon, the commission concluded that marijuana should be legalized or its classification downgraded to a much less restrictive classification of Schedule 4 or 5.[11] Nixon, being Nixon, decided to reject his own commission's findings, and cannabis remains a federal Schedule 1 drug to this day.

In 1974, Nixon formed NIDA (National Council on Drug Abuse) with a clear intention to only show detrimental effects from cannabis and other drugs, rather than expose potential medical benefits. Even today, funding for a NIDA research grant is *only* approved when attempting to show the *negative* effects from cannabis or other drugs.

Research scientists will tell you, accepted and supported scientific research methodology follows a process where a hypothesis is tested through unbiased methods (such as double-blind, randomized and placebo-controlled studies) to reach an unknown conclusion. Creating research only to support a previously determined and negative conclusion is just bad science.

The fight to keep cannabis in the hands of those who need it began almost immediately after its criminalization in 1971. Scientific support for the medical value of cannabis first emerged in 1976 with the court case of Robert Randall, a glaucoma patient who was steadily going blind at the age of twenty five. He was forced to fight his way through the court system in order to prove it was cannabis, and cannabis only, that was keeping him from going blind. Mr. Randall's marijuana was supplied to him by a government-owned facility located in Mississippi.[12] I discuss Mr. Randall's case further in Chapter 18.

The next battle for cannabis access was a direct result of the HIV-AIDS epidemic of the late 1980s and 1990s, which resulted in California legalizing access to cannabis with Proposition 215 in 1996. With this measure, cannabis was now legal on a state level but illegal on a federal level. All drugs are classified on both state and federal levels, so legalizing the use of cannabis on the state level still left users at risk of being arrested and prosecuted by the federal government. Currently, any state that has a legal cannabis program is a result of reclassification of the drug *on the state level*. I discuss this specific battle further in the chapter on HIV.

Why, with extensive scientific evidence supporting the medicinal value of cannabis, does our Federal Government still refuse to reclassify it to a less restrictive status, thus reducing legal penalties for its users and increasing access to those who need it? What *really* makes cannabis so "dangerous"? The answer is not based on safety and science but is deeply rooted in racism and money. Lots and lots of money!

In 2018, 62% of Americans believed cannabis should be legalized, yet it remains illegal on a federal level today while the rest of the globe acknowledges its medical value by incorporating it into their healthcare systems.[13] Politicians will tell you we need more scientific research. With the scientific research found in this book and others, this argument is antiquated at best. I think there is more likely something else motivating their political perspective, something with a lot of zeros at the end of it. It's really not that complicated: big money corporations (pharmaceutical, alcohol, and tobacco) have lost and will continue to lose, billions of dollars in business as cannabis is fully legalized. Forbes reported in 2018 that alcohol sales dropped 15% in states with medical marijuana laws.[14] That's *billions* of dollars in lost revenue every year.

Canada, France, Germany, and Spain are just a few countries that have adopted cannabis into their healthcare programs, so it is available to patients who need it. Why does the United States government refuse to do the same? One reason is the substantial power and influence wielded by Big Pharma. Over the last half-century, the pharmaceutical industry has established itself as the standard of treatment in the United States, and they have no intention of loosening that very profitable grip. Big Pharma will continue to be a patient's only option for medicine as long as cannabis remains federally classified as a Schedule 1 substance and the scientific evidence is ignored.

Pharmaceuticals Are Big, Big, Big Bu$ine$$

Pharmaceutical discoveries, such as antibiotics and insulin, have extended human life and decreased suffering for countless human beings over the last century. Drugs to reduce blood pressure and cholesterol have added decades to patients' lives with very tolerable side effects. Yet, somewhere along the way, the United States has become the most medicated country on the planet, spending more on healthcare than any other industrialized country in the world. Most countries spend about 5-10% of their Gross Domestic Product (GDP) on healthcare (United Kingdom 9.76%, Australia 9.25%, Japan 10.93%), yet the Unites States spends almost double that amount (17.09%) with a much lower life expectancy (United Kingdom #35, Australia #14, Japan #2, United States #43)[15,16]

A nice portion of those healthcare dollars goes directly into advertising. We are the only country besides New Zealand that allows for direct advertising of prescription drugs to patients. That's right, only two countries on the planet think it's a good idea to have pharmaceutical companies spend billions, literally billions, of healthcare dollars on advertising. If you watch television at all, you are inundated by their endless commercials on every channel. How is cannabis supposed to compete with these Goliaths that are intertwined with government agencies and funded by mountains of money? Cannabis advocates will tell you it's by taking one step at a time and never backing down. The legal battle to reschedule cannabis started immediately after Nixon made it illegal in 1970, and will continue until cannabis is available to all people who need it, thanks to organizations like NORML (National Organization for the Reform of Marijuana Laws). It's an uphill battle to resume access to cannabis, and patients have spoken; this multi- billion-dollar industry is not going away quietly.

There is a cozy, almost incestuous, relationship between the pharmaceutical industry and the FDA, the government agency in charge of approving new drugs and overseeing Big Pharma. The FDA can not reschedule cannabis, this must be done by the DEA or an Act of Congress, but the FDA is the authority when regulating cannabis or cannabis containing products under the Food, Drug, and Cosmetics Act. To date, they have been ambiguous about the role they need to take in the state marijuana market, but patients need their oversight to assure safe access to vape diluents and properly grown and tested flowers. Additionally, they can provide scientific evidence to affect the scheduling of THC, a molecule which is essentially identical to the prescription drug dronabinol (Marinol), a Schedule 3 drug. The FDA needs to stand up for the patients that use cannabis as their medicine in legal state cannabis markets.

Cannabis has been supplied to patients who need it from a government owned facility in Mississippi since the 1970s. How can the DEA and FDA administer cannabis to only a select group of patients who require it for life, then turn around and say that it holds no accepted medical value and they will not allow full access to cannabis for rest of the country? The legal arguments have been going on for decades and the insanity of it all is mind-numbing.

Fun fact: Money generated directly from pharmaceutical companies, in multiple arenas including fees for new drug applications, is what funds the oversight of the FDA. Big Pharma money funds the FDA. It's a bit twisted when you think about it and begs for corruption. This interwoven dynamic between the FDA and drug manufacturers can and has produced serious problems for consumers of medications in this country.

How the Opioid Epidemic Came to Life

An example of direct, negative consequences resulting from the relationship between the FDA and Big Pharma is the current opioid epidemic, which is ravaging the United States. 60 Minutes recently exposed how a long-acting opioid medication, OxyContin by Purdue Pharma, was approved in 1996 for use in patients for everything from back pain to post-surgical pain without a shred of scientific evidence showing that it was safe or effective for long term use, which is an absolute requirement for any drug approved by the FDA. Officials from Purdue Pharma said in depositions from a 2004 West Virginia lawsuit that the company did not hold clinical trials to show that OxyContin was less likely to be addictive or abused.[17,18] NO clinical trials, but FDA approval was granted anyway.

Previously, OxyContin had been approved only for short term use in cancer patients and for end of life care. With this single, scientifically unsupported decision by the FDA, they allowed the Sackler family of Purdue Pharma to aggressively market opioids at higher and higher dosages to anyone with pain, essentially creating generations of addicts while making billions for Purdue Pharma. It was unethical and disgraceful, and once exposed, the backlash against the Sackler family was swift and loud. After hundreds of wrongful death lawsuits were filed against Purdue Pharma, they recently declared bankruptcy. What responsibility does the FDA hold in this mess?

If this is how things continue to work in Washington, all patients will be forced to live under Big Pharma control for the foreseeable future without access to any alternative medications that are covered by insurance carriers. As mentioned on 60 Minutes and in the nationally bestselling book *Dopesick: Dealers, Doctors, and the Drug Company that Addicted America* by Beth Macy, an investigation into the opioid epidemic created by Purdue Pharma in West Virginia showed that FDA regulators—the people who are responsible for protecting patients against Big Pharma—are allowed to leave their positions at the FDA and head straight into high paying positions at the companies they were just in charge of regulating.[19,20] Talk about a conflict of interest!

The head regulator at the FDA responsible for practically creating the opioid crisis by allowing OxyContin to be prescribed for practically anything, Curtis Wright, went to work as a consultant for Purdue Pharma shortly after leaving his position within the FDA.[21] It is well known that once you leave the FDA, jobs await in the high paying pharmaceutical industry. The incentive to make decisions based on the possibility of a future in a lucrative market and with a grossly profitable company cannot be overstated. A non-compete clause in the work contract of FDA regulators would remove the ability to cross over between these industries and free FDA employees from scrutiny.

Big Pharma's Cannabis Epidiolex: Plant-Based, FDA-Approved CBD

In 2018, GW Pharmaceuticals, a pharmaceutical company based in Britain that also created a THC based drug called Sativex sold in Canada and the United Kingdom, was the first drug manufacturer to introduce a cannabis-based product to the American market when the FDA approved Epidiolex, a plant-based CBD solution indicated for treatment of seizures associated with Lennox-Gastaut syndrome (LGS) and Dravet syndrome (DS) in patients 2 years of age and older.[22] Epidiolex was approved by the FDA in June of 2018, *after* which CBD was reclassified from an illegal Schedule 1 substance to a benign Schedule 5 substance in September of 2018, as long as the product containing the CBD is FDA approved. How does a Federal 1 scheduled drug get approved by the FDA and *then* get rescheduled to a legal status? That sounds very expensive. And if it is appropriate for CBD, then why not THC? Why not whole plant cannabis?

If the CBD molecule (or any other cannabinoid) is held within the cannabis plant or a non-FDA approved tincture, like those sold over the counter under the Food, Drug, and Cosmetics Act, then that CBD is still technically illegal.[23] To add more confusion to the mix, a provision in the 2018 Farm Bill essentially legalized hemp in December of 2018.[24] Industrial hemp contains high amounts of CBD and less than 0.3% THC and is the main source of CBD for over the counter CBD products. Are you lost yet? I believe that's the idea.

Over the counter CBD products do not have the same regulatory oversight as prescription medications, and patients need to work much harder to find quality products that are made from reputable manufacturers. Also, these products, currently, are very expensive and their prices will drop substantially as cannabis is legalized, regulated, and companies have access to federally insured banks. Clearly, there is a high demand for CBD products and accurate, science-based information. If you keep people confused, they will simply stay with what they know, the "safe" pharmaceutical medications prescribed by their doctors.

Epidiolex will cost a patient without insurance at least $1,200 for 1000mg of plant-based CBD, another example of how companies are allowed to charge whatever they deem necessary with no restrictions on pricing established from the government. The cost of around 1000mg of CBD in a purified oil at a cannabis dispensary can cost a patient around $100, cheaper, but still out of reach for many who need it when not covered by insurance.

The issue when buying CBD in a dispensary is not necessarily safety, but a lack of consistency between products as well as the possible lack of availability. Both consistency and availability are not frequent issues when dealing with pharmaceutical products, but other problems do exist in the manufacturing process, most often performed outside the United

States. Recently a popular blood pressure drug, valsartan, was found to have cancer-causing impurities found in *millions* of pills manufactured in China.[25] In fact, most of the active chemical ingredients used in pharmaceutical medications are produced in China, a country *clearly* not regulated by the American government. With the cannabis industry in its infancy, standardization between formulas may be needed to facilitate a medical program, and I'm confident it will be established in the future as the cannabis industry continues to mature.

Does standardization between batches warrant a twelve-fold increase for a pharmaceutical product? We will have to wait and see. Price gouging by the pharmaceutical industry has become an accepted practice in healthcare and it needs to end. There has been a lot of talk on this issue with little action. Something stinks when Washington continually allows the sickest and weakest group of people in the country to support overbloated healthcare costs making pharmaceutical companies very, very wealthy in the process. Legalizing and regulating the cannabis industry will decrease costs for patients as insurance coverage kicks in, will allow access to federally insured banks (currently unavailable as a Schedule 1 drug), could generate billions in tax revenues, create thousands of jobs, and will pour money into our economy. None of this can happen as long as it remains an illegal Schedule 1 drug.

Is this who we have become as citizens of the greatest country on earth? I firmly believe in a capitalistic society, but above that I believe we have a moral and ethical responsibility to protect those who are most vulnerable, those with debilitating illness. I have been frustrated for decades by how our leaders force some patients to choose between their medicine and their next meal. As we discuss in upcoming chapters, it is possible that cannabis may actually be used to prevent many chronic, inflammatory diseases that cost billions in healthcare dollars.

There has been a systematic criminalization of cannabis for decades, but the end is in sight. Cannabis can be substituted for multiple pharmaceutical drugs, and that is a big problem for a massively profitable drug

alprazolam (Xanax)	pregabalin (Lyrica)	morphine	baclofen
diazepam (Valium)	duloxetine (Cymbalta)	oxycodone	methocarbamol
lorazepam (Ativan)	gabapentin (Neurontin)	hydromorphone	cyclobenzaprine
clonazepam (Klonopin)	amitriptyline (Elavil)	fentanyl	carisoprodol (Soma)
estazolam	nortriptyline (Pamelor)	methadone	dronabinol (Marinol)
flurazepam	desipramine (Norpramin)	meperidine	ondansetron (Zofran)
oxazepam	citalopram (Celexa)	buprenorphine	prochlorperazine
temazepam (Restoril)	escitalopram (Lexapro)	codeine	granisetron (Kytril)
triazolam (Halcion)	fluoxetine (Prozac)	acetaminophen (Tylenol)	dolasetron (Anzemet)
chlordiazepoxide (Librium)	fluvoxamine (Luvox)	ibuprofen (Advil, Motrin)	metoclopramide
clorazepate (Tranxene)	paroxetine (Paxil)	naproxen (Aleve)	megestrol (Megace)
diclofenac	sertraline (Zoloft)	dexamethasone (Decadron)	prednisolone (Orapred)
sumatriptan (Imitrex)	buproprion (Wellbutrin)	prednisone	acetazolamide (Diamox)
almotriptam (Axert)	eletriptan (Relpax)	frovatriptan (Frova)	naratriptan (Amerge)
phenobarbitol	carbamazepine	ethosuzimide	lamotrigine

enterprise. Do not believe the old hype and propaganda. The value of cannabis cannot be overstated. The time has come for cannabis to take its rightful place as a valid medical treatment.

The graphic on the previous page shows a sample of drugs that can be reduced or replaced with the use of medical cannabis.

Replacement of these drugs with cannabis translates into billions in lost profits for Big Pharma. In light of this, it's hard to give credence to the idea that it's not about the money.

CHAPTER 2

Understanding Cannabinoids and Terpenes

"In strict medical terms marijuana is far safer than many foods we commonly consume. For example, eating 10 raw potatoes can result in a toxic response. By comparison, it is physically impossible to eat enough marijuana to induce death. Marijuana in its natural form is one of the safest therapeutically active substances known to man. By any measure of rational analysis marijuana can be safely used within the supervised routine of medical care."

Francis Young[1]
DEA Administrative Law Judge

Scientists have presently identified over one hundred individual cannabinoids within the cannabis plant, THCA, CBDA and others, each with its own potential benefit for epilepsy, migraines, anxiety, pain, cancer, and more. A **cannabinoid** is simply a chemical molecule that acts upon a receptor, in this case, the receptors of the **Endocannabinoid Receptor System (ERS)**, just recently identified in the early 1990s.

Cannabinoids originating from plants are called "phyto-cannabinoids." These plant-based molecules work similarly to our own two "endo-cannabinoids," which are produced within our body in response to external stimuli. **Anandamide** (*ananda* is the Sanskrit word for bliss) is produced in the brain in response to stress and other factors, while **2-AG (2-arachidonoyl glycerol)** is thought to play an active role in regulating our circulatory system, offering a possible new target for the treatment of cardiac disease and diabetes.[2]

The ERS is woven throughout the brain and body and is an essential element for the maintenance of human health. Until recently, the ERS has not been a specific target for pharmaceutical therapies, but with cannabinoid science expanding, many believe modulation of the ERS is the future of medicine. The goal when using cannabis as medicine is to achieve a sense of balance, or homeostasis, which promotes physiological healing accompanied by a sense of peace and calm.

In this chapter, we shine a light on the science of cannabis with a focus on the:

- role of the endocannabinoid receptor system;
- major cannabinoids available in products sold in dispensaries (THC, THCA, CBD, and CBN) and their applications when treating symptoms of disease;
- process of decarboxylation, or activation, of a cannabinoid compound and what happens if we decide to skip this process and consume cannabinoids in the raw, plant form;
- role of terpenes; hydrocarbons that create the different smells of cannabis and offer unique medical characteristics.

I designed this chapter to help you understand how to apply the science of cannabis when treating disease. The following chapter will discuss how to specifically dose these molecules so they are comfortable, yet effective. By understanding the science of cannabinoids combined with dosing, you can gain the confidence you need when choosing your medicines at the dispensary. In addition, by understanding some basic cannabis terminology and forms of use, like how to use CBD and THC as an edible, you will begin to feel empowered when shopping for your medicine.

We begin with the ERS, the gateway for healing when using cannabis therapy.

The Endocannabinoid Receptor System (ERS) and Its Impact on Health

Cannabinoids are molecules housed in the beautiful crystals that cover the leaves of the cannabis plant and promote a chemical response through activation of CB1 and CB2 receptors of the endocannabinoid receptor system. We have multiple receptor systems throughout the body. For example, if you have pain, an opioid molecule (derived from the opium poppy flower) will attach to your opioid receptor (yes, that's what they are called), and the outcome is a decrease in pain felt throughout the body.

CB1 and CB2 receptors of the ERS are the most abundant receptors of any kind found throughout the body. They are found in high concentrations in the brain, spinal cord, and spleen but also have been identified in the eyes, skin, gastrointestinal tract and pancreas. The receptors of the ERS influence inflammation, pain, fear, the immune response, fertility, cardiac function, and blood pressure—almost every condition within the human body. I find it astonishing that the largest receptor system in the body, with the potential to affect dozens of diseases was not even discovered until the 1990s, but that's what happens when research is stifled by the government and profits are promoted elsewhere.

With cannabis still federally scheduled as an illegal drug, we are only just beginning to discover to what degree the endocannabinoid system influences our overall health. I follow a doctor from Canada on Twitter who reported using cannabis to successfully treat blood pressure and pulmonary hypertension. In fact, there are countless anecdotal reports all over social media on how patients use cannabis for everything from cancer to depression, but it's science and responsibly conducted research that legitimize cannabis within the medical community, as well as with patients, and determines when a drug will be covered by an insurance carrier.

Below is a list of responses generated through activation of CB1 and CB2 receptors of the ERS:

Endocannabinoid System Responses in the Human Body

emotions (acute and long-term depression)

memory

stress response

effects reproductive function

central nervous system

appetite

gastrointestinal activity

osmotic pressure within the eye

fat breakdown and synthesis

actions of diabetes (glucose metabolism in the cells)

cardiovascular system

inflammatory response

metabolism

pain response

There are over five hundred different molecules contained within the cannabis plant: including cannabinoids, terpenes, plant waxes, and flavonoids. For the purposes of this book, we are only going to focus on the top four cannabinoids currently available in cannabis dispensary products, CBD, THC, THCA, and CBN, as well as the most prevalent terpenes. I will also touch on CBC (cannabichromine) and CBG (cannabigerol) simply because I have found them in several over the counter CBD containing products and they offer significant medical benefits in their own right.

Trichomes

Cannabis is a visually beautiful plant, especially when viewed under the lens of a microscope. Google "trichome images" and you can quickly see the intrigue offered by the crystals, which coat the flowers of the cannabis plant and contain the bulk of its medical value.

Trichomes are resinous glands that blanket the buds (flowers) of the female cannabis plant. In nature, they protect the plant from predators and insects. For humans, they house the molecules that create the unique smells and effects of each individual cannabis strain.

The most abundant cannabinoid found in most strains of cannabis is THCA (tetrahydrocannabinolic acid). In the next section, I will discuss how THCA, the molecule found in the raw, cannabis plant, is transformed through decarboxylation into the active THC molecule (Δ-9-tetrahydrocannabinol) desired by most cannabis users.

CBD (cannabidiol) is the second most abundant molecule within most cannabis strains and is found in high concentrations in industrial hemp. CBD has received a lot of notoriety recently for its value in helping reduce epileptic seizures and helping patients with anxiety and pain. CBN (cannabinol) is not as well-known as THC and CBD but is available in products in both medical and recreational cannabis markets. Throughout the upcoming chapters, I will focus on these four cannabinoids and their applications for disease.

Decarboxylation of Cannabinoids: Activate!

When THC, CBD, and CBN are found in the raw form of the plant (inside the trichomes sitting on the leaves), they are in the acid form of the molecule. The acid form of THC, known as THCA, does not have euphoric or psychoactive properties. This means if you were to grab a handful of fresh cannabis buds and eat them without applying heat first, you would not experience a high feeling. If you read the chemical analysis on the label of any cannabis flower in a dispensary, it will show large amounts of the molecule THCA and low amounts of the molecule THC. I have helped many patients at the dispensary who were confused by the difference.

To activate the THCA molecule and transform it into the euphoric, medically active Δ-9-THC molecule, heat must be applied, which may be why people have smoked cannabis for centuries. Smoking is literally the easiest and fastest way to activate the cannabinoids and achieve the desired effect. According to the European Industrial Hemp Association (EIHA), "It would need 3 hours at 212°F (100 °C) to convert THCA fully into THC and 4 hours at 208.4°F (98°C). At high temperatures above 320°F (160°C) only about 10 minutes and at 392°F (200°C) only seconds are needed to convert THCA fully into THC."[3] Smoking heats cannabinoids to over 500ºF (260ºC).

Decarboxylation is the chemical process by which THCA is transformed into THC (or CBDA into CBD) as a carboxyl group is removed and carbon dioxide (CO_2) is released, but you may hear it referred to as "decarbing" when shopping in a dispensary. Cannabis flowers must be decarboxylated before the trichomes can be extracted and made into an edible. Smoking and vaporization of flowers heat and decarboxylate cannabinoids during the process of using them.

There is extensive information available on the Internet about how to properly decarboxylate your cannabis. (Greencamp.com is an excellent resource.) A simple method that can be performed in most ovens is to spread out the cannabis in a glass dish and bake it for 30 minutes at 240ºF. Decarboxylation performed in-home ovens can sometimes be uneven and patients can lose up to 20% of the cannabinoids in the process. If you don't trust your oven, the Nova Decarboxylator ($200 on Amazon) is a little device that allows you to get the maximum amount of cannabinoids out of your flower when making medicated edibles. Below is the chemical process by which decarboxylation occurs.

THC-A → heat → **THC**

Cannabinoids Available in Dispensaries

There may be over one hundred cannabinoids identified in cannabis, but only a handful are sold in high concentrations as products in dispensaries. Below are the most prominent cannabinoids currently sold in stores with some easy reference charts that list the basic medical applications for each molecule. Refer to these charts as often as needed. Most dispensary products include a blend of multiple cannabinoids rather than a single, isolated molecule. It is the ratio between cannabinoids which will influence the overall feeling and effect. For example, products rich in CBD with lower amounts of THC are often better tolerated by new cannabis patients since CBD helps to reduce the euphoria of THC.

In the next section, I will discuss how to apply these cannabinoids to specific diseases. Looking toward the future, it is likely that new cannabinoids will be added to the marketplace. For example, recent reports discuss how growers are looking for ways to increase the amount of CBG (cannabigerol) in strains, a cannabinoid shown to be effective for combating inflammatory bowel conditions as well as glaucoma.

THC (Δ-9-tetrahydrocannabinol) is available in inhaled, sublingual, oral, and topical products and has dose-related euphoria. (The more you take, the stronger it feels.) Select dispensaries carry THC nasal sprays (used for epilepsy), low dose suppositories, and topical patches.

THC is most often used for pain, nausea, depression, anxiety, insomnia, migraines, and to reduce muscle spasms, but it holds great potential in fighting cancer and beyond.

THCA (Δ-9-tetrahydrocannabinolic acid) is available in select medical dispensaries as oral products only (tincture and oils) and is of great interest to researchers since in most respects it is identical to THC, but being in the acid form does not have psychoactive properties. One study revealed that THCA may be more potent than THC in reducing nausea.[4] If you're looking to reduce THC euphoria in cannabis therapies, consider trying THCA products. Begin with a very low starting dose, such as 1mg every 8 hours, and increase the dose slowly as discussed in the next chapter.

CBD (cannabidiol) is available as inhaled, sublingual, oral, and topical applications. In cannabis dispensaries, CBD is frequently paired with THC for its synergistic effects when looking to reduce pain and when used to relieve side effects of chemotherapy. If the CBD dose in a product is at least twice as high as the THC dose, the psychoactive effects from THC become milder and more tolerable.

CBD sold over the counter is sourced from industrial hemp and is identical to CBD found in all other strains of cannabis. Products that are sold outside cannabis dispensaries may, or may not, have additional terpenes, discussed momentarily, and cannabinoids added to them that will enhance the overall wakeful or sleepy effects of the final product.

Medical benefits of CBD hit the mainstream media with the discovery of their use in controlling seizures in children. It is currently being studied for use with brain injuries, such as Chronic Traumatic Encephalopathy (CTE), an injury most often associated with football players and boxers. CBD is a potent anti-inflammatory, and its use has been established for general pain management, decreasing acute nerve pain, anti-tumor, seizure control, mild anxiety, and sleep. When you think of CBD, think of a potent anti-inflammatory with mild to moderate pain relief.

CBN (cannabinol) is available in products such as Mary's Medicinals and Kikoko Tranquil-Teas, as well as undiluted, CO_2 extracted oils and tinctures in select dispensaries. CBN is derived when THC naturally degrades over time due to light and heat, so it may have mild hallucinogenic properties, although most patients I speak with say there is no euphoria. CBN has shown potential for reducing pain and inflammation, which may help with conditions such as arthritis, nerve damage, and migraines.[5]

CBG (cannabigerol), specifically CBGA, is the chemical parent to both THC and CBD. Specific enzymes, along with light and heat, interact with CBGA to form THCA and CBDA, along with a third cannabinoid, CBCA. Breeders are attempting to influence this chemical reaction in order to produce strains high in CBG for its inflammation reducing qualities in the eye (glaucoma), gastrointestinal tract, and brain. Research has shown CBG to have antibacterial activity against methicillin-resistant Staphylococcus aureus (MRSA), a deadly skin infection, too.

CBC (cannabichromene) is a non-psychoactive cannabinoid that is available in many strains of flowers as well as over the counter CBD formulations. CBC can help decrease pain and inflammation and increase the body's production of anandamide. Researchers are interested in its possible benefits for cancer, irritable bowel syndrome, Crohn's disease, acne, neuropathy, and chronic post-operative pain because it seems to work synergistically with other cannabinoids.

Cannabinoid Applications (THC, CBD, CBN, and THCA)

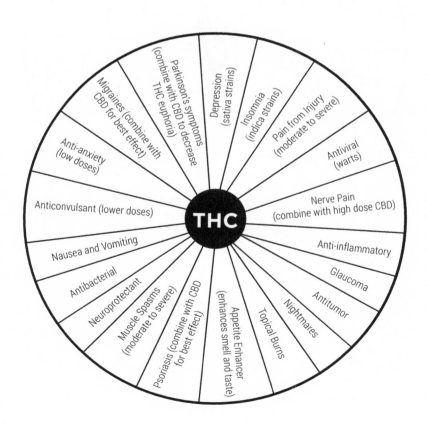

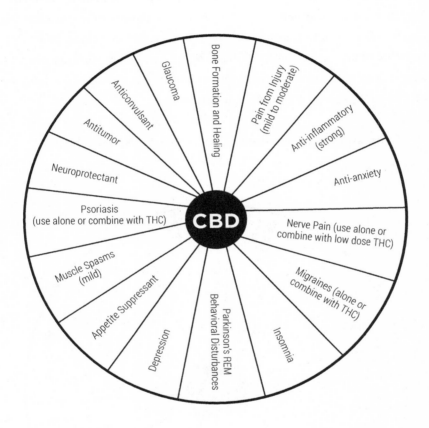

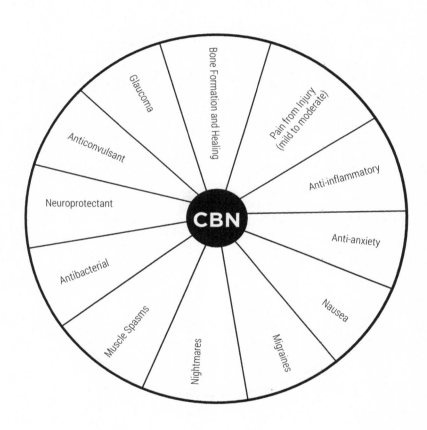

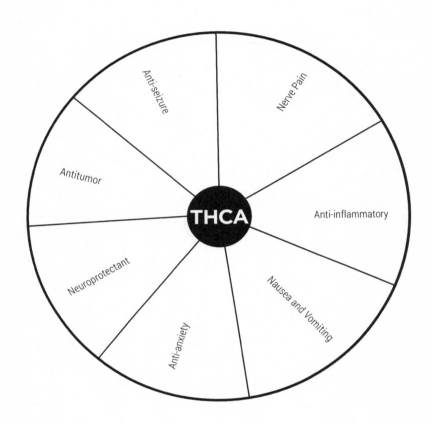

I realize that this is a lot of information all at once, but don't let it overwhelm you. Refer to these charts as often as needed until you learn how to effectively use each cannabinoid, just as you learned how to take each of your prescription pills.

You might be wondering how you'll be able to know which cannabinoids will work best for you. In reality, cannabinoids seem to work best and feel most comfortable when used together, as found in the natural whole plant. CBD can help the psychoactive side effects of THC feel less pronounced and THC can work synergistically with CBD to decrease pain and anxiety. Again, it is all about the ratio between the two molecules.

As with any drug, the only way to know how it will affect you is to try it. If you are a patient who has been using opioids for months or years to treat your pain, I bet you can tell me how quickly the pill will begin working, exactly how long it will last, what withdrawal symptoms feel like and every conceivable side effect. Cannabis is simply another drug. In this case, we focus on the effects when cannabinoids (THC and CBD) are used separately and when combined together. In the next chapter, we discuss the specifics of delivering a comfortable dose of each cannabinoid.

Before you actually try anything, I'm going to walk you through what's available in most cannabis dispensaries and offer recommendations for how to get started based on your symptoms and comfort level. Let's say that your issue is pain. (We discuss pain in detail in Chapter 8.) In the chart above, you can see that all cannabinoids seem to work for pain, so where do you start? And how? Do you inhale or take an edible?

The quick answer is: There is no wrong place to start, except by starting with too much THC. Consuming excess THC as a new cannabis user could make you never want to try it again. When beginning cannabis therapy, start where *you* feel most comfortable. If you are a bit hesitant to try THC, simply start with a product rich in CBD with very little to no THC. It will be helpful to know what time of day to use an indica or sativa strain, discussed momentarily, but other than that, there is no wrong answer as to where to begin. When looking for the best result, pick a comfortable starting point and plan for adjustments as described in the next chapter.

As you can see from the previous chart, CBD works for almost every medical condition in this book (except nausea) and has no high feeling, which makes it an ideal entry point when starting cannabis for most patients who may be nervous about using THC. The effects will change a little by adding a little THC and will change dramatically by adding a lot of THC. I discuss this process in detail in Chapter 3. When starting with CBD, follow the guidelines in the next chapter to help get the most out of the molecule. If you decide you want to just smoke a little cannabis and see what happens but are afraid, follow the guidelines under inhalation to ensure a comfortable beginner's experience.

Cannabis has a lot of components, so let's focus on just these four molecules (CBD, THC, THCA, and CBN) as your medicine. Use them alone or together; it's up to you. There is no wrong product to start using. My goal is to help you get the most out of each product you purchase. It is not a single-step process, and as with any new medication, will require adjustments.

Once you become comfortable with the applications of each cannabinoid, you can begin using your products for issues you previously never would have considered. You might use THC for a sunburn, CBD for psoriasis, or CBN for stress. The next chapter will discuss how to initiate the dosing of each molecule to create a comfortable experience and will focus on how to apply them to specific disease symptoms. Remember, the goal is to feel great, and there is no wrong way to use cannabis unless of course, you take a bit too much. Even if you do over consume, know you are safe, the cannabinoid effects will wear off and you will be just fine.

The Prescription THC Pill: Why Not Just Get That?

A synthetic, laboratory made THC isomer is available by prescription under the drug name dronabinol (brand name Marinol) and does not contain any additional cannabinoids or terpenes normally found from plant-derived THC. Marinol was listed as a Schedule 2 drug (like oxycodone) upon approval by the FDA in 1985 with labeling indications for appetite stimulation and nausea relief. (Although it may be tough to keep a pill down when nauseated.)

In 1995, the drug manufacturer UNIMED petitioned the DEA to reschedule dronabinol, once again, to a less restrictive Schedule 3 substance. This was approved in 1999, and dronabinol, a substance almost identical to THC, remains a Schedule 3 substance to this day.[6] This puts it on par with testosterone and many cough suppressant medications.

While consulting with new cannabis patients who have tried dronabinol, I inquire as to what caused them to stop taking their pills and turn to cannabis instead. Patients often state that they felt strong psychotropic side effects even when taking the smallest dose of dronabinol available or they complained that the pills were all together ineffective when attempting to stimulate appetite or stop nausea.

For some patients, the high cost of the pills is a factor. When the brand name Marinol was the only product available, a monthly prescription of just sixty pills would cost over $500. Today, the generic can still cost close to $400 for the same sixty pills. With high deductible insurance plans being the norm, many patients cannot afford these high prices for an anti-nausea drug. If we were to compare the price of the synthetic THC pill to plant-derived THC available in dispensaries, the plant-derived THC is seven to eight times lower in price than the dronabinol available in pharmacies with the added benefit of natural terpenes and additional cannabinoids. It's also been shown that patients who are dealing with nausea and vomiting find inhalation a more effective delivery method than oral delivery.

I attribute some of the lack of efficacy with the synthetic THC pill to a lack of additional terpenes, flavonoids, and cannabinoids that naturally occur in whole-plant cannabis oils and contribute to the overall medical effect. This is known as "the entourage effect." With the synthetic THC pill, there is a single molecule in a sesame oil base, and it has not been shown to be as effective as natural cannabis for either appetite stimulation or for decreasing nausea and vomiting. Whole plant cannabis is more comfortable and effective than the isolated THC molecule and patients are better able to control their individual dosage.

The Entourage Effect

When molecules work synergistically, as they do in whole plant cannabis, we get a phenomenon called the entourage effect, a term first coined by a group of scientists in 1998 that included "the father of cannabis research", renowned Israeli biochemist Dr. Raphael Mechoulam.[7] Aristotle was the first to define synergy as the whole being greater than the sum of its parts which definitely applies to cannabis.

Secondary cannabinoids, such as CBG, CBDV, THCV, along with plant terpenes and flavonoids, significantly influence the overall medical effect of each cannabis strain, including the strength of euphoria from THC and whether a strain brings about wakefulness or sleepiness. The entourage effect is well summarized on the website ProjectCBD.org, a non-profit group that offers current research and guidance about CBD and cannabis. I frequently refer to their research studies and appreciate their dedication to cannabis science.

The Role of Terpenes

THC and CBD, the two most abundant cannabinoids found in most strains of cannabis and our primary focus in this book, provide much of the medicinal effects of cannabis products sold in dispensaries, but there are more players in this game that influence the overall *feeling* and outcome of each individual cannabis strain. If you try a sativa flower one day and the next day try an equally potent indica flower you can immediately identify the difference. This is due to the terpene content.

Terpenes are fragrance hydrocarbons produced in several varieties of plants, not just cannabis, and contribute to the physical effect of each strain. Terpenes' biggest contribution is whether a strain will get you up and moving or knock you back into bed. They may also exhibit some influence on a strain's effectiveness when treating nausea, anxiety, pain, and depression.

Terpenes have medicinal properties in their own right. For example, linalool is best known for the floral odor it gives to lavender and has been used to induce relaxation and as a sleep aid for centuries. The smell of citrus in fruit comes from limonene. It has been traditionally used to reduce symptoms of anxiety and depression.

Here, we focus on the eight most common terpenes found in the most abundant concentrations tested in cannabis today. This doesn't mean you need to memorize the terpene list before every visit to the dispensary. An easier and more pleasurable way to learn about terpenes is to take note of which terpenes are found in the highest amounts of strains you enjoy and document the information in your journal. If a patient is familiar with terpene effects, such as through the use of aroma-therapy oils, they can base their cannabis choices solely on the concentration of the terpenes.

Below is a chart that shows the common sources of the most prevalent terpenes found in cannabis. Certain fragrances will feel more familiar and comfortable to your senses, and I recommend following your instincts. One gentleman at the dispensary searched for high concentrations of alpha-pinene (think Pine-Sol cleaner), which helped open his lungs to breathe easier. Another patient had a severe allergy to lemons and needed to avoid strains very high in limonene or she would begin to itch all over her body. Observe which terpenes you love and which you might want to avoid. If you taste a strain and absolutely love the flavor and effect, write it down in your journal so you can be sure to pick it up again during your next trip to the dispensary.

	Found in	Used for	Aroma
Linalool	Lavender	Sleep and relaxation Anxiety Pain	Floral
Terpineol	Oregano Marjoram Cumin Lilac	Antitumor Antibacterial Anti-fungal Insomnia	Floral (lilac) Anise Mint
B-Caryophyllene	Black Pepper Cloves Thai basil	Antibacterial Anti-septic Anti-inflammatory Antitumor	Spicy
Humulene (isomer of beta-caryophyllene)	Hops Sage Coriander	Inflammation	Earthy Hops-like
B-Myrcene	Mango Hops Bay leaves Eucalyptus	Anti-tumor Anti-inflammatory Spasms Insomnia	Earthy Fruity Clove-like
A-Pinene	Pine trees Orange peels	Bronchodilator Asthma	Pine
Limonene	Lemons Oranges	Stimulates the Immune System Anti-fungal Gastric Reflux	Citrus
Borneol	Teak Family of Trees	Coughs and Cold Pain Swelling	Camphor Mint

This chart is meant to be used as a guide only. I do not recommend consuming isolated terpenes to treat disease without the advice of a doctor because certain terpenes are safe in small amounts, but others, such as borneol, become toxic if swallowed in large quantities.

Indica, Hybrid, and Sativa Strains

Terpenes, along with certain physical characteristics of the cannabis plant, help determine whether a strain will be classified as an **indica, hybrid, or sativa**. These three terms are probably the most important to understand before you begin shopping for cannabis. If you understand the basic differences between the terms indica and sativa, you are halfway to becoming a cannabis expert. (Well, that may be a bit of a stretch, but it's a start.) I can make this incredibly easy:

Cannabis **Sativa** (sa-ti-va) is **sunny** (sunny sativa) and is, therefore, for daytime use to wake you up (the sun awakens).

Cannabis **Indica** (in-di-ca) puts you **in-da-bed/in-da-couch**. These strains relax the body and can put you to sleep (depending on the terpene profile).

For most cannabis users, a sativa strain will be used during the daytime for energy and focus while indica strains are used for relaxation of both the body and mind. These indications may not apply to every user. I have patients who use indica strains throughout the day for epilepsy or anxiety, so consider this a general way for new users to categorize strains of cannabis.

A hybrid strain is typically a man-made creation. It is created when a grower crosses two distinct strains of cannabis to form a new unique strain. Theoretically, new strains of cannabis with new effects are being created every day, a very exciting concept. When crossing a sativa and an indica strain (very popular), the outcome is something that falls in between a sativa (very stimulating) and an indica (very relaxing), which many people enjoy. Hybrid strains that lean on the sativa end of the spectrum are called **sativa-dominant hybrids** and are appropriate for people who deal with both depression and anxiety. Hybrid strains that lean on the indica side of the spectrum are called **indica-dominant hybrids** and can be effective for increasing appetite, decreasing anxiety, and for after work when you may want to relax but not necessarily go to sleep. The best way to determine if you like a sativa or an indica strain is to try it.

While doing research for this book, I discovered the naming system that has been used for the cannabis genus for the last forty years is technically incorrect. Botanist Richard Evan Schultes, the man who created the original taxonomy for cannabis in the 1970s, misidentified Cannabis afghanica as Cannabis indica. Patients new to using cannabis are already overwhelmed with information, so I do not want to create any more confusion. But I found the story interesting and think you may too. If you are interested, check out my blog post about it on my SwayInnovations.com for more information.

I recently helped a patient navigate the dispensaries in New York State and was disappointed by the lack of natural, isolated cannabis terpenes found in the products. Sadly, the state vetoed cannabis flower for their medical program, which resulted in dispensaries exclusively extracting oils for their products. The oils are blended, and individual terpene profiles are lost. The intrinsic medical value of the terpenes was ignored by the state legislature, an enormous detriment to the patients as well as the growers. The beauty of cannabis is not in the isolated cannabinoids. This kind of thinking follows a pharmaceutical model and needs to be avoided. Cannabis in all its varieties offers endless choices, so patients can find the best strain for their specific problem. What they have done in New York is remove the ability to find patient-specific strains and, maintaining a one size fits all mentality.

Hemp Oil versus Hemp Extract versus Phytocannabinoid-Rich Hemp Oil (PCR)

Over the counter CBD products are becoming increasingly popular, and many patients ask me to analyze the CBD products they've purchased at various stores and online. As a pharmacist, the first thing I do is flip the box over and read the list of ingredients. I was often confused because some products say hemp oil, some say hemp extract, others say CBD oil or PCR. I discovered that there are significant differences between these products:

1. **Hemp oil** is derived from the seeds of the Cannabis *sativa* plant, also known as hemp. None of the plant material is used when making the product. Seeds contain no CBD or THC, but are rich in certain oils, including omega oils. These products may have certain health benefits, but do not contain CBD or THC and therefore will not work as an analgesic or to decrease anxiety.

2. **Hemp extract** is derived from the whole hemp plant (Cannabis *sativa*), also known as industrial hemp, which contains high amounts of CBD and less than 0.3% THC. Hemp extract, sometimes called CBD oil, does contain the compound CBD and may even contain other non-psychoactive cannabinoids such as CBG, CBC or CBN. These products do not contain THC.

3. **PCR** is the latest ingredient listed in over the counter supplements and several brands of pet treats. PCR, or **phytocannabinoid-rich hemp oil**, includes the molecule CBD along with other beneficial compounds found within the hemp plant such as terpenes and flavonoids. These products do not contain THC.

I find the labeling for CBD and hemp containing products confusing, so I can't imagine how the average person goes about navigating the CBD market without professional assistance. When shopping for an over the counter CBD product, only purchase products manufactured in the United States from companies that use the best manufacturing process and utilize the input of pharmacists and other scientists. Do not grab a bottle at the gas station. At best it may be a complete waste of money, and at worst it will contain dangerous ingredients.

Products may or may not have additional ingredients added to help with insomnia or pain, so read your labels carefully. I have found products sold in stores that include additional cannabinoids like CBG and CBN. These cannabinoids can add medical benefits to the overall effect without a high feeling. Over the counter products never include the psychoactive molecule THC because these products are only available in recreational and medical cannabis dispensaries.

SECTION 2

Consuming Cannabis

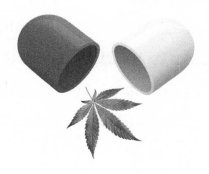

Eli Lilly, Parke-Davis
(now owned by Pfizer) and Squibb
of Bristol-Myers Squibb all sold
multiple medical marijuana
products at the turn of
the 20th century.

CHAPTER 3

How to Consume Cannabis Safely, Comfortably, and Effectively

"Not only can cannabis work for a variety of conditions such as epilepsy, multiple sclerosis and pain, sometimes, it is the only thing that works. I changed my mind, and I am certain you can, as well. It is time for safe and regulated medical marijuana to be made available nationally."
Dr. Sanjay Gupta[1]
CNN.com Chief Medical Correspondent

By now, you have a general understanding of the differences between an indica (sleepy), a hybrid, and a sativa (wakeful) strain, as well as the common medical applications for THC, CBD, THCA and CBN, the most prevalent cannabinoids found in any cannabis dispensary. Refer to the previous chapters again and again as you experiment and learn about your new products.

Once you understand the functions of each cannabinoid, it's time to learn how to dose them effectively and comfortably. Proper dosing is always a critical component when administering medication. This chapter will clearly explain how to start using cannabis by inhalation, sublingually, or as an edible. Proper utilization of all cannabinoids, especially THC, can mean the difference between feeling fantastic, feeling nothing, or feeling uncomfortable.

When the first dose of an edible or even a vaporizer is too strong, patients can feel dejected and may believe cannabis is not right for them. This may be true, but the problem is more likely resolved by an adjustment in dosage, trying a different strain, or sampling a different delivery method.

As millions can attest, getting "high" is easy. Take a big dose of THC and boom, you're high. But, in my experience, medical patients don't want to escape life by being high all day, rather they just want to feel better and be more productive. Less pain, fewer migraines, less anxiety, and a sense of wellbeing is the overall objective. This chapter will help you get there. Relax, and remember, it's ok if you accidentally consume too much cannabis. Take it slow, document your progress in a journal, and you just may find the kind of relief that everyone is raving about.

Take it Low and Slow

The number one rule when starting cannabis therapy is to begin with a small, specific dose of your cannabinoids and increase the dosage slowly and systematically until maximum efficacy is established with minimal side effects. Taking more of any drug is not necessarily better; it's just more. Aim to find *your* best dose by listening to your body. This is personalized pharmacy.

Cannabis has a "sweet spot" in dosing where optimal benefits are observed, and side effects are comfortable. There are no established dosing guidelines for cannabis, and this can make things confusing for new patients.

Try to be patient when learning to use cannabis. Patients who feel sick often want to rush the process to feel better quickly, and this is totally understandable. Most patients who start using cannabis find significant relief within a few days, but others may require a bit more time and need more guidance. If you have found some relief but are starting to feel overwhelmed at the process, feel free to contact me at my website SwayInnovations.com for additional instruction.

Recently, a doctor friend on Twitter posted regarding a patient with malignant hypertension (blood pressure above 180/120mmHg) who used a 1:1 (equal THC and CBD) medical cannabis oil and was able to discontinue all pharmaceutical hypertension medications. Very exciting stuff! The problem is that no exact dose could be given so other patients could follow suit. This is because cannabis must be tailored to each patient and does not fit the one-size-fits-all drug concept.

When medicating with a pharmaceutical drug, your dose is based on the results of a small clinical trial and may not be optimal for your body, your race or your gender. The ability to find your best dose of cannabis requires more work than popping a pre-measured dose in a pill, but that is an asset when treating symptoms, not a detriment.

Document your progress in a journal. It can be hard to remember the details of your experience because cannabis can affect your short-term memory, but several recent studies, including the "Review of the Neurological Benefits of Phytocannabinoids" published in Surgical Neurology International (2018), demonstrate the neuroprotective properties of THC as well as CBD, so use your products knowing you are helping, not hurting your brain.[2] Excess THC consumption can lead to a serious lack of motivation, increased anxiety, and contribute to weight gain (thanks to "the munchies"), but the claim that using cannabis harms your brain is pure Anslinger propaganda.

Because each cannabis strain has unique characteristics, document negative and positive side effects in your journal. Does a certain strain give you a headache every time you use it? Write down its name and terpene profile for future reference (although these effects may also be due to nutrients used when the plant was grown). Does a strain make you unable to stop eating everything in the pantry? Write it down. You may want to skip that strain if you need to lose weight. Cannabis is meant to work for you, not against your goals.

Drug Interactions with Cannabis

Cannabis is a complex plant that contains hundreds of molecules that contribute to its overall effect. The more drug molecules that are consumed simultaneously, the more likely a drug interaction can develop.

Most drugs are metabolized in the liver, and if many drugs are placed in the body at once, it's only natural that something could happen.

Before June of 2018, we had little scientific data regarding drug interactions between cannabis and pharmaceutical medications. Dronabinol (Marinol), the synthetic THC isomer pill, lists a few minor drug interactions and has been on the market since 1985, meaning that if a compelling drug interaction did exist, it would have made itself known in the last thirty-five years.

With the approval of Epidiolex, a cannabis-derived CBD solution approved for seizure disorders, we get the chance to see how a plant-based CBD molecule interacts with other pharmaceuticals. The non-profit group Real of Caring (theroc.us), located in Colorado, provides an easy to read reference chart of drug interactions between CBD and anti-epileptic medications, a class of drugs frequently prescribed with CBD to reduce seizure activity and well known to have frequent drug interactions in their own right. I refer to the information provided by the Real of Caring often and recommend that you check out their website for the latest clinical studies. (They do not offer medical advice.)

In studies conducted on liver isoenzymes (the place where interactions most occur), CBD was found to have minor interactions with CYP1A1, CYP1A2, CYP, 1B1, CYP2D6, CYP3A4, and CYP2C19, the most significant of which is an interaction with CYP2D6.[3,4,5,6,7,8,9] If an enzyme metabolizes two drugs at the same time, the potential for a drug interaction exists. In practice, drug interactions can often be identified relatively quickly by physicians when monitoring a patient and their blood work. Doctors and pharmacists monitor blood work all the time for a variety of reasons, and when liver enzymes become elevated it can be indicative of a problem that needs to be addressed.

A good example of this process is when St. John's Wort, an herbal supplement used for treating depression, became popular in the 1990s. Doctors and pharmacists quickly noticed how it strangely began to affect people's heart medications. The drug interaction was studied and published, and today is well established and documented so patients taking certain cardiac drugs can be warned to avoid St. John's Wort.

Cannabis was legalized in California in 1996 followed by Oregon, Alaska, and Washington in 1998.[10] Even with people keeping their cannabis use to themselves, I believe a significant drug interaction would have been discovered in the last thirty years.

For instance, patients with HIV are very likely to use cannabis and HIV drugs together, drugs with frequent and well-established drug interactions, yet no problems have been reported regarding HIV drugs combined with cannabis. Is it really possible that everybody in medicine—pharmacists, doctors, and nurses—have simply missed important drug interactions between HIV drugs and cannabis over the last fifty years? I think it's more likely that cannabis has minor drug interactions, rather than significant issues with the majority of currently available pharmaceutical drugs. Clearly, well funded clinical trials are required for additional discovery.

Here are the current facts regarding drug interactions with CBD and THC (redacted from the FDA drug package insert of dronabinol and the Epocrates drug reference app):[11]

1. There are severe drug interactions listed for both CBD and synthetic THC (dronabinol) with a drug called clobazam (Onfi, Sympazan), an anti-seizure drug used for a childhood seizure disorder called Lennox-Gastaut Syndrome. Clobazam is not a widely prescribed medication due to toxic side effects.

2. As previously mentioned, CBD has a minor inhibition of several liver enzymes with one enzyme listed as a moderate interaction (Epocrates app). Minor drug interactions typically do not call for a change in medication but should be monitored during therapy by your prescriber.

3. Synthetic THC, dronabinol, has no drug interactions listed on Epocrates, my favorite medical drug information app.

The bottom line is that cannabis use by adults is on the rise, and we are not seeing a sudden increase in reports of serious drug interactions with commonly prescribed drugs like statins, cholesterol-lowering medications known to have numerous drug interactions. This can change as new drugs enter the market. In medicine, doctors and pharmacists know to look for trouble with certain classes of drugs when taken together: anti-fungals, blood thinners, digoxin, and macrolide antibiotics, for example. These drugs have well established and frequent drug interactions where therapies often need to be adjusted.

If you are a patient who takes medication, especially multiple medications, I recommend informing your doctor about your cannabis consumption so they can monitor your liver enzymes and blood work for abnormalities. If you have a doctor who is against the use of medical cannabis, it may be time to find a new doctor. It is always better to be informed than in the dark. If something looks unusual, your doctor can take action. Cannabis has over four hundred compounds, so realistically we may never have a comprehensive list of pharmaceutical drug interactions. However, we will develop a better understanding of this issue as the body of scientifically derived knowledge grows.

What's to Buy in a Cannabis Dispensary?
Most Common Products Available

People new to using cannabis can quickly become overwhelmed by the number of products available in a cannabis dispensary—vapor cartridges, pre-rolls, edibles, tinctures. Wow! Where is a person supposed to start?

Look at the variety of products as a bonus rather than a bad thing. Start with the delivery method you feel most comfortable with and branch out from there. The upcoming sections will inform you on how to start using cannabis whether you start with a puff or a gummy candy. Eventually, you will find your favorite. There is no right or wrong answer. Remember, when using cannabis, you are free to sample different items to find what suits you best, which is what makes it so appealing to so many people. Most people find that they prefer to have access to a variety of products than being restricted to just a few.

Dispensary Products Typically Available

Inhaled Products: cannabis flowers, oil cartridges, and concentrates

Sublingual Products: oils, tinctures (alcohol based products can not be used sublingually), sublingual sprays, film strips

Oral Products: edibles, oils, tinctures, pills, capsules

Topical Products: creams, lotions, balms, oils

In addition to the products listed above, some dispensaries carry topical patches and nasal sprays (for epilepsy), but these products are not widely available in all markets. Refer to your dispensary's website, browse their menu, or give them a call if you are looking for a specific product.

Patients starting cannabis therapy often have preconceived notions of which delivery system they will prefer before they have actually tried it. Several patients I have counseled had no desire to inhale anything and were only interested in edibles, but as I explained the differences in timing between the different delivery methods, they began to realize that edibles may not be best for their symptoms. Other patients require the long-acting effects of an edible to get through the night. Most patients prefer a variety of products. For example, some use edibles along with inhaled products depending on the time of day they are medicating and the severity of their symptoms. I simply ask you to be open-minded. What's best for you may surprise you.

Timing Is Everything When Medicating

The first aspect to understand when medicating with cannabis is the **duration of action** for the drug. How long before it starts working, and how long will the effects last? The different delivery systems do not have the same onset or duration of action, so it's important to understand the differences. Understanding how to time your cannabis dose will allow you to plan your day and medicate effectively to avoid overconsumption.

Inhalation works fast, but the effects are usually short lived and will require patients to medicate more frequently when treating nausea or pain. Edibles and oral products can take 1–2 hours to begin working, which may not be ideal if you are nauseated or in severe pain. Sublingual timing is somewhere in between inhaled and oral timing.

Higher doses of all delivery methods may last longer than lower doses and will feel stronger, so try to avoid overlapping doses. Medicate, wait an appropriate amount of time, and re-medicate if needed. If you re-dose too quickly, you risk becoming overly inebriated and drowsy. Timing is everything in life and cannabis is no exception.

If this sounds complicated simply try a puff or an appropriate dosage of an edible, follow the directions coming up, and it will all come into focus.

How to Medicate by Inhalation (Smoking or Vaping)

The primary advantage when medicating by inhalation is that it works almost *instantly*. Imagine that your tremors, anxiety, nausea, or pain could vanish within seconds to minutes of taking your medicine, and you could easily increase your dose if needed.

For patients suffering from chronic pain, certain days, especially cold, rainy days, lead to increased levels of pain, yet patients are not allowed to increase their daily prescribed opioid dosage. Because cannabis has very low toxicity, the limitations in dosing as seen with opioids and other pharmaceutical medications do not exist. If you have a day with more pain, more nausea, or more anxiety, feel free to take another puff or two or three. A little extra dose can equate to a lot more relief.

Let's be clear, *inhaling* does not equate to "smoking" in reference to cannabis. The biggest complaint among new cannabis users is they do not want to smoke anything, much less something that will immediately draw attention to themselves. Smoking cannabis produces a strong, identifiable odor, which for many people is undesirable. No worries. Smoking is not necessary to medicate with cannabis when using inhalation. I will share more about how to smoke and vaporize (as well as equipment needed) in the next chapter.

For now, when a drug is inhaled, molecules are rapidly absorbed into the bloodstream through millions of tiny blood vessels called alveoli. The lungs are frequently used to deliver medication because they contain a large surface area appropriate for quick drug absorption. Drugs delivered to the bloodstream through the lungs do not pass through the liver, a process called "the first-pass metabolism." Avoiding the liver provides a more predictable response than if the medication were swallowed, as it would be when consuming an edible. The patient receives a rapid, predictable response within seconds to minutes. If you have ever used a rescue inhaler (albuterol) for asthma, you understand how quickly the drug resolves tightness in the lungs and helps patients breathe easier fast.

When medicating by using inhalation, follow the directions below in order to avoid overconsumption. There is no need to be nervous, just inhale one puff at a time. If you accidentally overshoot and consume too much just wait anywhere from 15 minutes to an hour for the effects to wear off.

Inhaled a bit too much? You just learned what it feels like to consume too much THC. (It happens to everyone at some point.) As you become more experienced with using cannabis, consuming too much THC is more of an annoyance than anything else. There is absolutely no danger, so just try to relax.

Timing Inhaled Doses

Breathe in slowly 1 puff (2-3 seconds in duration) maximum. Do not keep inhaling or you risk over consumption.

You will feel the effects within 1-15 minutes.

If the dose is too low, re-medicate with 1-2 puffs after 20 to 30 minutes.

Effects from inhalation last from 1-3 hours. Medicate as needed.

How to Medicate by Sublingual Administration

Sublingual administration of cannabis oil is an excellent alternative to inhalation for patients who do not like, or simply can't, inhale properly but who need a relatively fast acting product to treat their symptoms. Like inhalation, sublingual doses deliver higher blood drug levels than oral routes because cannabinoids are delivered directly to the bloodstream and do not go through first-pass metabolism in the liver.

Products start working within 5–20 minutes when applied under the tongue or between the cheek and the gum (called buccal dosing), slightly slower than when medicating by inhalation. Under our tongue and on the side of the cheek are thousands of tiny blood vessels that help medications quickly absorb into the bloodstream for a fast, predictable response.

Nitroglycerin is an example of a sublingually administered drug that's been used to treat angina since 1876.[10] It is available in sublingual dissolving pills and sprays just like cannabis products and relieves chest pain within 5–15 minutes of administration.

It is important that you not place a sublingual product on top of your tongue because you will swallow it, making it work like an edible. Sublingual products offer a discreet way to medicate, which is preferable for many patients that need to medicate around the clock.

Sublingual or buccal dosing should be used when patients are:

1. unable to inhale and need rapid relief,

2. unable to absorb medications through the stomach,

3. or unable to swallow medications.

Timing Sublingual Doses

Apply under the tongue or between cheek and gum. Do not eat or drink for 10–15 minutes after dose.

You will notice the effect within 5–30 minutes.

If the dose is too low, re-medicate after 3 hours.

The effects of sublingual products can last 3–4 hours.

If accidentally swallowed, sublinguals work like edibles, so be sure to place under the tongue or between the cheek and gum.

You'll find more about the most common sublingual products available in dispensaries in Chapter 5.

How to Medicate with an Edible (Orally)

Edibles, or oral formulations of cannabis, have become extremely popular within the expanding cannabis industry for their long-acting effects and yummy delivery systems. Patients who are not educated about the correct way to consume an edible can unintentionally devour more than needed setting themselves up for an uncomfortable experience that can last for several hours.

The most common mistake made by patients unfamiliar with cannabis edibles is to assume, usually about 30 minutes after taking an edible, that it is not strong enough, so they take another one only to realize about 2 hours later that the first dose was, in fact, more than sufficient.

Oral delivery is ideal for patients combating around the clock symptoms and can work as a preventative measure for conditions such as migraines, chemotherapy side effects, and Parkinson's disease symptoms. Patients who consistently medicate with the same dose around the clock tend to notice that they develop a tolerance to the psychoactive effects of

THC. If you take the same dose of THC, around the same time every day, it won't feel as strong as taking a single dose of THC only once or twice a week.

As previously mentioned, when cannabis is swallowed it is absorbed through the gastrointestinal tract and undergoes first-pass metabolism in the liver. This substantially decreases the amount of medicine available in the bloodstream. Metabolism through the liver creates a less predictable response than inhalation or sublingual administration, meaning, one patient can find an edible takes forty-five minutes to start working while another patient can discover it takes two hours.

Bioavailability is the extent to which a nutrient or medication can be used by the body. Research has shown only 4–20% of an oral dose of cannabis will be available in the bloodstream versus bioavailability between 31-56% when administered by inhalation.[11, 12]

Besides a low bioavailability, when cannabinoids are absorbed from the oral route of administration, drug onset varies greatly from patient to patient. This unpredictability in dosing pushes some patients to medicate with inhaled products over edibles exclusively. I find most people notice edibles begin working 45–60 minutes after consumption, although for a smaller number of patients it can take up to two hours. Using a journal and following the instructions below regarding how to dose THC and CBD will help you learn how edibles work in your body. A big meal can delay the onset of action, so consuming cannabis on an empty stomach can help edibles work a bit faster. The base into which the edible is made can affect the onset timing as well. For instance, a liquid product may have a faster onset than a dense brownie.

In rare circumstances, I have spoken with patients who feel no effect when using oral cannabis products. This can be due to a very high tolerance or variances in liver enzymes. If this is the case for you, medicate with inhaled or sublingual products exclusively. I discuss available edibles in more detail in Chapter 6.

Timing Edible Doses

Take with a small amount of food but not on a full stomach, or the effect will be delayed.

Liquid products will work slightly faster than foods.

Onset is between 45 minutes and 2 hours.

Do not re-dose for 6 hours, especially if this is your first time taking an edible.

Edibles last from 4–12 hours depending on the patient. Most patients experience the effects of edibles for 4–6 hours.

Higher and excessive dosages can last longer than lower dosages, so it is important to find your most comfortable and effective dose.

How to Comfortably Begin Using THC

THC is the most abundant molecule in the majority of cannabis strains and the molecule most likely to cause problems for people new to medicating with cannabis. THC causes **dose-related euphoria**, meaning, a little will produce a mild effect while a lot will produce a strong effect. If you have used cannabis before and did not enjoy the experience, it may simply be an issue of ingesting too much THC when a lower dose or one mixed with CBD would have been more pleasurable.

When designing a THC treatment protocol, patients should slowly and systematically increase their dosage until they feel it is comfortable and effective. THC sensitivity differs drastically between patients. I have seen one person who could barely consume 2mg of THC comfortably while others can take 100mg and go for a 2-hour hike through the mountains. The rule of thumb is to start low and take your time. Once you know "your numbers", they don't tend to change.

If you already consume prescription medications that cause substantial drowsiness or dizziness, combining these with THC can exacerbate these side effects. If you reduce or remove these medications once you determine cannabis can be effective for your symptoms, you can better titrate your dose to experience optimal relief with substantially less drowsiness. Talk to your doctor or visit my website as to how to reduce your pharmaceutical medications safely and effectively. It is important to include your prescriber in the process.

Inhalation

As mentioned, when using products containing THC alone or combined with CBD (in close to equal amounts), begin with 1 puff only. *Do not* inhale deeply for longer than 2-3 seconds or you risk consuming too strong a dose. The effects of inhalation are fast, so wait at least 20 minutes before re-medicating. Cannabis flowers can differ in their THC concentration by over 15%. (That is a lot!). So, some products may be substantially stronger than others. If you begin using every product with just 1 puff every 20–30 minutes, you can safely determine the strength of a product within minutes without becoming overly intoxicated.

Sublingual

Tinctures are frequently used for sublingual dosing because they act fast and provide an easy way to administer THC at a very low and specific dosage. Make sure you are familiar with how many milligrams (mg) are contained in each milliliter (ml) of your product (more on that in Chapter 5), so you can slowly and confidently increase the amount of THC over time.

THC should be started at a dose of 2–3mg and placed under the tongue or between the cheek and gum. (Remember, not on top of your tongue.) If sensitive to medications, begin with as little as 1mg. Sublingual effects last 3–4 hours. Increase your THC dose by 2–3mg about every 24 hours, *not* every dose. Although, if you begin using 2–3mg and feel absolutely nothing, wait 4 hours and increase your dose by another 2–3mg (total of 5mg) of THC immediately. If feeling overly drowsy (sativa products included), try dosing less often, every 6 to 8 hours, or decrease your dose by 25% and reevaluate. High doses of THC *will* cause excessive drowsiness.

Oral Dosing

THC is available as edible products in recreational dispensaries in increments of 2.5–10mg. Stronger products are available in medical markets. New patients should begin with 2.5mg of THC or less. If you are unsure or nervous, begin with only 1–2mg for your first dose. Only consume what makes you feel comfortable and adjust from there. You can usually achieve lower doses with liquid formulations.

Do not re-medicate for at least 6 hours to determine how quickly the THC will begin working in your system and how long edibles work for you. Write the effects down in your journal.

Increase the dose of THC by 2.5mg every 24–48 hours—not every dose—although if you feel absolutely nothing with a dose of 2.5mg THC, increase the next dose to 5mg after the first 6 hours and remain at 5mg for at least 24 hours. You want to feel something, but do not continue to increase your dose too quickly or it can be harder to "dial-in" the dose. Be sure to document your progress.

If a dose felt good but a bit too strong, you can either decrease the dose by 25% or combine your dose with at least *double* the amount of CBD. The more CBD to THC, the milder the euphoria of THC will feel, so if you want a very mild THC effect, try taking 10mg of CBD with 2.5mg of THC (a 5:1 ratio) or higher. Once again, if you feel tired or drowsy, decrease the THC dose by 25% or wait a longer period of time between doses.

Negative Side Effects of too Much THC

Negative side effects of THC can occur when the dose is too high. Patients can experience anxiety, nausea, vomiting (at very high doses), rapid heartbeat, muscle weakness (including falls), confusion, hallucinations, extreme dizziness, and extreme drowsiness. These are dose-related side effects, meaning that if you consume just a little too much THC you may just feel a little anxious while consuming a lot of excess THC can cause patients to feel paranoid or even vomit. Follow the instructions given in this chapter and this will not happen to you. Taking THC with equal or higher amounts of CBD will feel different and is often preferable for many patients, especially during the daytime. Patients that prefer to combine THC with higher doses of CBD describe feeling more clear-headed and comfortable.

If you do accidentally consume too much THC, here are some tips to help alleviate the effects until they can wear off:

1. If you have a prescription medication such as a benzodiazepine that's intended for anxiety, take one dose only. This may help with THC-induced anxiety. The combination may cause excessive drowsiness, however, so plan for a nap. Do not consume a benzodiazepine if you have consumed alcohol or opioids within the last 4 hours.

2. If you do not have prescription anxiety medications, take 25–50mg of diphenhydramine (Benadryl), which may also cause excessive drowsiness.

3. If you have CBD in an edible form with *no* THC, take at least twice the milligrams of CBD that you took THC. For example, if you took 10mg of THC and it feels too strong, take 20–30mg plain CBD. If you are not sure of how much THC you took, try a dose of 40–50mg of CBD.

4. If you have CBD in a vaporizer (again, *no* THC), inhale five strong puffs (or more).

5. An old trick to decrease the psychoactive side effects of THC is to crush black pepper corns and slowly and gently breathe in the aroma through your nose. In addition, you can chew on one or two whole pepper-corns.

---

6. Have a snack, preferably something with a small amount of sugar or carbohydrates.

7. Take a shower or bath. Warm water can be very comforting.

8. Call a friend. Having someone tell you things will be okay can be very helpful when your mind wants to call 9-1-1.

9. Go to bed. Put on some meditative music and try to go to sleep.

10. Move your body. High doses of THC can feel physically uncomfortable. Try doing some yoga or going for a walk in familiar surroundings or clean your house. Keep the tasks simple. Don't try to do your taxes. Stay in a place where you are comfortable and feel safe. And remember, this *is* going to wear off!

Effectively Dosing CBD

CBD is excellent for treating pain, anxiety, and inflammation, but its effects can feel mild and may not be effective for patients dealing with more severe symptoms. I encourage patients new to cannabis to first try CBD products that contain little or no THC to see how they compare to products that contain more THC. More often than not, the greatest benefit of cannabis is seen when using a combination of cannabinoids because of the entourage effect mentioned earlier. Remember, isolating molecules comes from a pharmaceutical model. Blends of multiple cannabinoids frequently feel the best.

The biggest problem when using over the counter CBD oral products is using a dose that is sub-therapeutic and turns out to be just a waste of money. Most people will need a minimum of 10 mg dose of CBD to feel the effects. It can be difficult to determine an effective dose when using CBD by inhalation, so just go by how you feel. Like THC, oral doses of CBD should be started low (5–10mg) and increased **every three to five days** to find the sweet spot of effectiveness. CBD works differently than THC and you need to take more time when dialing in your dose.

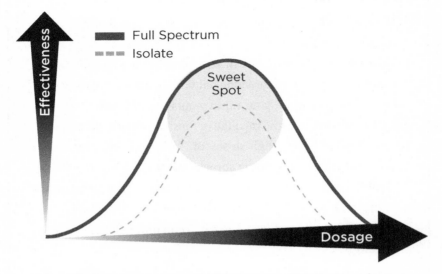

Full Spectrum CBD vs CBD Isolate

CBD has a **bell curve dose-response** where lower and higher dosages have the least effectiveness and the most effective dose is somewhere in between. Whole plant, or full-spectrum, cannabis, most often found in dispensaries, has a bigger effective area under the curve than isolated CBD formulations found in many over the counter products, but you can still find an effective dose when using these products.

When treating chronic conditions such as pain, repeat the dose every 6–8 hours around the clock, although heavy pain days may require dosing at 4 hours intervals. It can take several days to observe optimal benefits from your CBD treatments, so take your time and only increase the dosage every 3 to 5 days. Too low a dose will be ineffective and too high a dose will give unwanted side effects (and be less effective). Listen to and trust your body.

Products containing CBD *only* or with very little THC (a ratio of greater than 10:1 CBD:THC) do not have psychotropic side effects. The closer the ratio approaches to equal amounts of THC and CBD the stronger the THC will feel.

CBD Oral Dosing

10mg every 4 to 12 hours

Increase by 5–10mg per dose every 3 to 5 days.

Stop increasing your dose when negative side effects occur

(listed below) or no additional benefit is observed.

Negative Side Effects of CBD

The most common dose-related side effects from CBD are a mild headache and abdominal cramping or discomfort. Also listed as side effects for Epidiolex are sedation, sleepiness, and decreased appetite. So, you may want to avoid CBD if you want to increase your appetite. Like THC, these side effects tend to be dose-related and may be eliminated by decreasing the dose of CBD by 25% or more.

Dosing with Cannabinol (CBN)

Most new cannabis users aren't familiar with cannabinol, but it may offer unique benefits for conditions such as pain, inflammation or anxiety. CBN is formed as cannabis naturally ages and THC degrades to form the CBN molecule. In my experience, patients find CBN to be relaxing, with applications for anxiety and sleep disorders, but quality clinical studies are required to determine the full range of medical effects. When using CBN, begin with 1–2mg every 6 to 8 hours and increase every 24 to 48 hours by 1–2 mg until happy with the effects.

Micro-Dosing

Micro-dosing is a process in which patients use very small, sub-therapeutic dosages of THC (with or without CBD) to achieve health benefits without becoming inebriated. Micro-dosing has become increasingly popular with LSD and other psychotropic drugs to enhance creativity, energy, and focus.

THE CANNABIS PRESCRIPTION

Patients can micro-dose using all delivery methods: inhalation, sublingual, or oral. For inhaled products, inhale one puff every 6–8 hours throughout the day. If the effects are not sufficient, increase the dose to 2 puffs or continue to use one puff more frequently, perhaps every 3–4 hours. The goal is to reduce your symptoms and build your tolerance without becoming intoxicated and tired.

For sublingual or oral dosing, begin with as little as 1mg of THC taken two to three times a day (every 8–12 hours). Increase the dose *very* slowly by as little as 1mg every 5–7 days until the most benefit is experienced.

	Inhalation	Sublingual	Edible
Starting Dose	Take one (2–4 second) puff.	Take 1mg of CBD and THC.	Take 1mg of CBD and THC.
Frequency	every 6 hours	every 8 hours	every 8–12 hours
Increasing Dose	Increase number of puffs or frequency until effective.	Increase by 1mg of both THC and CBD every 5 to 7 days.	Increase by 1mg of both THC and CBD every 5 to 7 days.

Effective micro-doses can be as little as 1–2mg per dose or up to 10mg for patients who have developed a substantial THC tolerance. Occasional dose increases may be needed when an illness spikes or during increased times of stress, but generally people aim to take very low doses around the clock to keep the body in a state of homeostasis without intoxication.

Are you feeling a bit overwhelmed by it all? I truly hope not. When cannabis is applied as medicine it can be a lot of information to process at once, but I promise that if you follow these steps for how to begin medicating with your chosen product, things come into focus very quickly.

Learning to use cannabis requires a little bit of knowledge combined with patience. If you throw caution to the wind, as some people do when using recreational cannabis, and brazenly consume too much THC, you are going to pay the price and never fully achieve what you really want, which is to just feel better. Respect the plant. Take your time. The goal is to feel relaxed and comfortable with a reduction in symptoms. Millions upon millions of people have successfully used cannabis to find relief and so can you.

By the end of the 20th century, more than 20 prescription products that contained cannabis could be found on pharmacy shelves across the United States.

CHAPTER 4

Vape versus Smoke

"I grew up knowing that cannabis could be a medicine ... I'm not aware of any proven long-term [harmful] effects from cannabis. People have been trying to find major risks [from marijuana], but I've never seen any documented. We know if you smoke cannabis your chances of getting lung cancer are less than if you don't smoke anything at all."
David L. Bearman, MD[1]
Physician and Medical Marijuana Expert

When asked, most people will equate smoking cannabis to smoking cigarettes. Both produce smoke that is inhaled into the lungs, so it's not a stretch to assume both will cause damage to the lungs over time. But, science does not support this conclusion. A 2006 study funded by the National Institute on Drug Abuse (NIDA) and conducted by Dr. Donald Tashkin, a pulmonologist at the University of California Los Angeles who has spent over forty years studying the effects of cannabis on the lungs, concluded that smoking cannabis does not lead to lung cancer.[2] As we know now, this same outcome cannot be expected when smoking tobacco. Dr. Tashkin's conclusion has been supported by a twenty-year study (March 1985–August 2006) that followed over five thousand participants and concluded that low to moderate cannabis use did not adversely affect lung function.[3]

Even with this information, most new patients are not going to want to smoke cannabis. As discussed in the previous chapter, inhalation is a valuable method of delivery for cannabinoids due to its rapid absorption and fast-acting effects and because it gives patients the ability to achieve precise dosing. For patients who do not want to smoke but who need the fast action offered by inhalation, vaporization of both flowers and cannabis oil are alternatives that deliver all the benefits of cannabis without actually combusting plant material in the process.

In this chapter, I discuss the equipment needed for smoking and vaporizing cannabis flowers as well as vaporizing cannabis oil. We'll look at how "cannabis oil" is made, the diluents used in oil vapor cartridges, and substances to avoid in products available in today's market.

Oil vapor cartridges have become very popular within the cannabis industry for their ease of use and lack of odor, but an absence of regulatory oversight means manufacturers can use cheap and unhealthy fillers that can severely harm patients. Never, ever purchase black market cannabis cartridges, as the makers of such products have no concern for your health. Finally, I will provide a few tips on the proper way to inhale in order to deliver a suitable dose.

How Flower Products Are Sold in a Dispensary

It takes a lot of love, care, and patience to get the mature cannabis flowers from the plant onto dispensary shelves. Growers must harvest the buds at just the right time and then dry and cure them to enhance cannabinoid concentrations, develop terpene profiles and reduce harshness within the final product. Proper drying and curing also allows the buds to be stored for long periods of time without developing mold or deteriorating and reducing the cannabinoid concentrations.

Cannabis flowers should be stored in a dark, cool, and moisture-controlled container. Keep temperatures below 78°F (25°C) to avoid mold growth and degradation of cannabinoids. **CV Vaults** are a type of humidor and are standard in the cannabis industry. The top of a CV vault holds a natural salt packet that keeps the humidity between 58 and 62%, perfect for your beautiful buds.

If you prefer to have several cannabis strains on hand at all times, you can buy a few small vaults ($25 Amazon) that hold up to a 1/2 ounce (14 grams) in each container. Once the salt packet becomes dry and hard, they can be replaced for a few dollars. CV vaults seal tightly but do not contain a locking mechanism and should, therefore, be placed in a safe or locked cabinet along with all cannabis containing products. Keeping your medicine out of the wrong hands (kids or nosy guests) is imperative and will require vigilance.

Dispensaries sell cannabis buds or flowers in several units of measure as well as "pre-rolls" (aka joints). There may be a cost saving when purchasing larger quantities of flower, so check how your dispensary sets their prices.

When trying a new strain, I recommend purchasing the smallest quantity available to sample before investing in a larger amount. Be aware that plants do sell out, so if you love a particular product do not hesitate to buy more immediately and store it properly. If you invest in a large quantity of cannabis flowers, do yourself a favor and store it in a humidor.

Weighed Cannabis Flower

Dried flower sold in dispensaries is ready to smoke or vaporize. It's available for purchase by the gram or quarter, half or full ounce and only needs to be ground or broken up before using. Hard, dense buds do not burn properly. A "grinder", sold in most dispensaries, can be used for this purpose.

Ounces	1/8 ounce	1/4 ounce	1/2 ounce	1 ounce
Grams	3.5 grams	7 grams	14 grams	28 grams

Pre-Rolls or "Joints"

Pre-rolls are what most people know to be a "joint" with a paper filter on the end and can be used for multiple medicating sessions. As a new cannabis user, inhale a puff or two and put it out! Pre-rolls are not like tobacco cigarettes. Unlike cigarettes, which keep burning, pre-rolls tend to go out if not being continually smoked. People new to using cannabis often assume you need to smoke the whole thing. Not true! Medicate with an appropriate dose (one or two puffs to start), and put it out until the next time you need it. You won't regret your decision.

What Exactly is Kief and Hash?

The leaves and stems of cannabis flowers are not required for medicating. Cannabinoid rich trichomes can be extracted to be used alone in a more concentrated (stronger) product. Kief and hash are two products produced when trichomes are removed from the leaves.

Trichome extraction is done through several methods. The simplest and oldest extraction technique is to place the dried and cured cannabis buds in a container covered with a fine mesh screen. Simply shake, shake, shake the container, and the trichomes will fall off the leaves of the plant through the screen where they can be placed into a glass container.

Once collected, the trichomes without the leaves are called *kief*. This product can be smoked or vaporized by itself, used to make butter for edibles (decarboxylate, add to oil, and you're done), or sprinkled on top of cannabis flower to increase its potency.

If you apply heat and pressure to kief, you can form what's known as *hash*. Both kief and hash are concentrated flower products and have a much stronger effect than when using cannabis flower alone.

Equipment for Smoking Cannabis

Smoking marijuana occurs when you burn the flowers (buds) in a pipe or rolled paper, inhale, and hold for a few seconds before exhaling comfortably. The idea that you need to inhale and hold your breath for as long as possible is a myth and a harmful one at that.

Cannabinoids pass into lung tissues very quickly after inhalation. If you continue to hold the smoke in your lungs, you are allowing unneeded tar and toxins to absorb into them. Smokers only need to hold the inhalation in their lungs for a very short period (about 3–5 seconds) to allow the cannabinoids to enter the bloodstream.

Pipes

Besides pre-rolls, pipes are one of the easiest ways to smoke cannabis. Instruments used for smoking cannabis can literally be made from anything: glass, wood, stone. Fruit has even been used to smoke cannabis. A quick search of YouTube will yield many videos showing you how that's done.

Most inexpensive pipes for smoking are made of glass. The quality of the glass is often reflected in the price. I recommend using a pipe that is large enough to allow for adequate cooling of the smoke but not so large that it is hard to hold. The smaller the pipe, the closer your mouth and lungs will be to the flame, so it will feel hot and harsh while inhaling. Consider pipes that are a minimum of 4 to 5 inches or longer.

When using a pipe, place a small piece of loose plant material on top of a metal screen (available at dispensaries) to avoid inhaling the generated ash. A "carb," or carburetor, controls airflow and requires only about two minutes of practice. Cover the carburetor when lighting the plant material and begin inhaling. Uncover the carb when done lighting the cannabis as you continue to inhale.

Over time, pipes become coated with a dark, sticky resinous material and need to be cleaned with an alcohol-based product. Cannabis resin is not soluble in water but is soluble in alcohol (and oil). There are several pipe cleaning products on the market that do a great job. Some patients prefer to put their glassware in the dishwasher, but I have never tried this method for cleaning.

If you want to smoke but don't want to use a lighter, there are electronic smoking devices available such as the MegaToke XL ($349). This device combusts flowers and can be used for concentrates (coming up) as well. Patients simply load the device with ground flower and hit a button. Simple!

Water Pipes (Bongs)

Water pipes are another popular way of smoking cannabis because they filter the smoke through water, which both cools the smoke and removes ash produced in the burning process. If you want to keep your expensive glass water pipe pristine, you can purchase an **ash catcher**. Ash catchers attach to the pipe and do exactly what their name says: They keep ash and resin from reaching the water pipe, thus keeping expensive smoking devices clean and beautiful.

Some ash catchers contain a percolator device that will diffuse the dense smoke to create a smoother inhale. If you want to cool and smooth the smoke even more, add ice cubes to the water or place them in the tube of the water pipe.

If you are like every person who has ever owned a water bong, you will, on at least one occasion, knock it over and spill the stinky water all over your floor. Look for glassware with a large, solid base to increase stability and change the water frequently. All equipment used for smoking cannabis should be cleaned regularly.

Three Methods of Vaporization

There are three different methods of vaporization available in today's cannabis market, which creates a lot of confusion for people new to cannabis. While many vaporizers use only one method (flowers), some vaporizer machines can be used to vaporize both oil concentrates and flowers. A simple change of the oven in the device is all it takes.

Flower Vaporizer

Flower vaporization uses flower material that is typically ground and placed in the oven.

Oil Vaporizer

Oil vaporization occurs when a cartridge containing cannabis oil is attached to a battery that heats up the oil until it vaporizes and is inhaled.

Wax (or Concentrate) Vaporizer

Wax or concentrate vaporization uses thicker, more concentrated forms of cannabis oil such as wax, shatter, or budder. These products vaporize at higher temperatures than oil cartridges and require a hot surface, typically called a "coil" or a "nail."

As previously discussed, **combustion** occurs when smoking the plant material. This process will leave you with a pile of ash upon completion. Vaporization of the flowers restricts temperatures to below 500°F. This vaporizes the trichomes alone while leaving behind dried out plant material that looks like dead, fall leaves. Smoking raises the temperature of the cannabinoids above what is required to produce a vapor, so, essentially, you are burning away your medicine.

Temperatures used for vaping should be above 320°F (160°C) and below 465°F (240°C).

THC begins to vaporize at 315°F (157°C) and is destroyed at over 500° (260°C).

THCV evaporates at 428°F (220°C).

CBD evaporates between 320°F (160°C) and 355°F (179°C).

CBG requires temperatures above 390°F (200°C) to evaporate and offers maximum release at around 445°F (230°C).

Conduction versus Convection Vaporizers

Vaporizing cannabis is not a new concept, but some of today's vaporizers are more akin to a smartphone than a smoking device. **Conduction** vaporizers force heated air *over* the flower while **convection** vaporizers apply heat directly to the flower, which can give a stronger, denser vapor. Which vaporizer is best for you is a matter of personal preference. These days, most flower vaporizers are reviewed on YouTube which can help

Top Conduction Vaporizer	Top Convection Vaporizer
DaVinci IQ	Volcano
Pax 3	Firefly 2
Arizer Solo 2	Plenty

you decide which vaporizer best suits your needs and budget.

Begin medicating at a low-temperature setting, and experiment with the different settings as you get to know your new device. Be sure to clean your vaporizer regularly with specially designed cleaning solutions for cannabis devices (usually alcohol-based). There are numerous video tutorials available on the Internet for how to use and clean cannabis vaporizers.

How to Use a Vaporizer

- Grind or break up cannabis flower so the maximum amount of trichomes will be exposed to heat. Large, hard, dense buds will not vaporize effectively.
- Load the vaporizer, but do not overfill it. If the vaporizer is packed too tightly the air cannot flow through the oven.
- Turn the vaporizer on.
- Allow the vaporizer to reach the set temperature (lower temps are best for flavor).
- Inhale *slowly*. A strong, fast, hard inhalation will cause the device not to work properly.
- Inhale a comfortable number or puffs (one to two if unsure).
- Turn off the vaporizer when you're fully medicated or increase the temperature by one setting.
- Inhale a comfortable number of puffs at the higher temperature.
- At this point, you may cycle through the heat settings or continue medicating on the low-temperature settings. Higher

temperatures will produce a denser, sometimes harsher, puff.
- Halfway through a long treatment session, open the oven and stir the ground cannabis to expose all the trichomes to the heat.
- Close and continue medicating.
- You do not have to finish the entire contents of the vaporizer. Save remaining product for your next session, although the flavor will not be as good as if would be if it were fresh.
- When the device no longer produces vapor, turn it off and let it cool.
- Empty the dry, "already vaped bud" (AVB) into a glass container if you're planning to extract its contents further to make edibles or tinctures. Otherwise, simply throw it away.

Portable versus Tabletop Vaporizers

Vaporizers are available in handheld (portable) or tabletop models. If you plan to use vaporization as your primary method of medicating, I encourage you to buy a high-quality vaporizer with a good warranty.

The Volcano (three year warranty) and the Herbalizer (two year warranty) are the top of the line tabletop vaporizers. Each unit costs over $500 but is well worth it. Both digital models can vaporize flowers and concentrated oils beautifully and consistently.

I was introduced to the Easy Vape Digital tabletop vaporizer (no warranty) more than fifteen years ago, and it still holds its value today. This model, with its simple features, costs under $90 but offers patients precise temperature control and good reliability.

Portable vaporizers range from simple (Kandy Pens, Herb-E, Mig Vapor, and AtmosRx) to devices designed for the technologically savvy (PAX and DaVinci). More and more devices are introduced every year, so do your research to find one with the features that are most important to you.

If you are anything like me, you want simplicity and reliability. I like

PAX vaporizers because they work well and come with a ten-year warranty. The Khan Vaporizer has a quick heating time and a long battery life while the Pulsar APX V2 is a good option for under $100.

Do you like the idea of filtering the vapor through water for a smoother inhale? The Hydrology9 vaporizer by Cloudious9 ($199) is a portable vaporizer with an innovative design that cools the vapor with water while retaining the flavor of the cannabis.

Depending on your device, you may see white vapor when you exhale. This is not smoke, and it will not smell like cannabis smoke. The odor is sometimes described as burnt popcorn, but it will not identify you as a cannabis smoker. Higher temperature settings will provide a denser vapor.

If you decide vaporizing is right for you, be sure to clean your vaporizer regularly and keep it charged. It's a sad moment when you come across a dead battery right when you need to medicate.

Definition of "Cannabis Oil"

The term "cannabis oil" is ubiquitous in a dispensary. Cannabis oil is used to make just about every product found in a dispensary including vapor cartridges, edibles and capsules, topical balms, and concentrated extractions called concentrates/shatters/butter/waxes/caviar/live resin. For the purpose of this book, I am going to use the term "concentrate" when referring to the group of concentrated oils that contain THC greater than 70% (not for beginners!). Cannabis flowers contain THC content between 1 and 33%, a wide range of strength, yet still much lower than concentrates.

When making oil, trichomes are removed from the plant with the use of a solvent. The most common solvents are alcohol, butane, or highly pressurized CO_2 molecules.

In the recreational market, butane or butane-like solvents became popular for cannabis oil production because the extraction can be done with almost no expertise, and the required equipment is inexpensive.

There are two important issues to consider with butane extraction: first, the final product may have butane residue in it, and, more importantly, butane extraction is highly flammable. Many explosions have occurred while making **butane (BHO) cannabis oil**.

Large manufacturers of cannabis oil use **supercritical CO_2 extraction** machines, which use highly pressurized CO_2 molecules to extract cannabinoids and terpenes. Once the oil is extracted, any remaining CO_2 molecules simply evaporate, creating a "solvent-less" extraction process and a pure final product.

Extraction using alcohol followed by heat was perfected by Rick Simpson, who created the famous **RSO (Rick Simpson Oil)**. The final product is a dark, thick oil that contains decarboxylated cannabinoids along with every molecule held within the plant. Patients use these highly concentrated oils both orally and topically. I will cover undiluted RSO in more detail in Chapter 7.

Rosin is a type of plant resin produced when cannabis flowers are pressed between two heated plates. This process produces a beautiful, sticky oil full of terpenes, waxes, lipids, and cannabinoids. "Pure pressure half Lb of herb into 60 grams of rosin" is a professionally performed rosin extraction you can watch on YouTube.[4] For patients who wish to produce their own pure cannabis oils, NugSmasher and Rosin Tech Products offer rosin makers designed for home use.

As you can see, "cannabis oil" does not have a single definition. Extracted oils are initially highly concentrated and must be diluted when used in vapor cartridges for new cannabis patients. Up next, we discuss all the different products that can be made from extracted cannabis oil.

Concentrates/Wax/Shatter/Budder/Live Resin/Rosin/Dabs/Sauce

Concentrated oils contain very high levels of cannabinoids, specifically THC and CBD. These oils are sold under a variety of names based on physical factors of the final product. A **shatter** is hard like peanut brittle while a **sauce** has a more soupy consistency. Concentrated cannabis oils have potencies above 70% THC and can go as high as 96% THC (very strong!). They are available in CBD dominant strains as well. It is nearly impossible to establish a low dose of a concentrate, so new or low tolerance users beware. One puff of a concentrated oil can equal 1/2 to 3/4 of a whole joint. Yes, you heard that right, almost a full joint inhaled with just one strong puff of a concentrated oil.

Concentrated oils, although very strong, do not contain artificial diluents as found in oil vapor cartridges and are, therefore, preferred by cannabis purists who don't want to consume anything other than cannabis in their products. **Concentrates** are vaporized using a "wax," or concentrate vaporizer, which heats the oils at a higher temperature than used for oil vaporizer cartridges. For more advanced cannabis users, a glass or silicone "rig" is used. A **rig** is similar to a bong, but specifically designed to be used with concentrated oils. MassRoots has a great video tutorial on YouTube called "How to Take a Dab" if you are interested in what happens during the dabbing process.[5]

With an **oil rig**, a small drop of oil is placed on a very hot surface (called a nail) where it's immediately vaporized and inhaled. For patients who require a high dosage, concentrates are an efficient way to medicate. Try to keep temperatures as low as possible to protect delicate throat and lung tissues.

Pre-filled Vapor Pens (no Additional Battery Required)

Oil vapor pens look like an electronic cigarette and may just be the easiest products in the entire dispensary to use. Pens are pre-loaded with diluted cannabis oil and require no additional battery; just remove from the package and inhale slowly. Pens will turn off after the dose is administered, but if you need more just inhale another puff.

Dosist pens were a Time Top 25 invention of 2016.[6] They are available as six proprietary blended formulas that have "no additional fillers." The pens have names like calm, sleep, relief (for pain), and passion. A three second inhale administers an exact dose of 2.25mg. The best part of a Dosist pen is their recycling program. Return an empty Dosist pen to any retailer and receive $5 towards your next Dosist purchase.

Dosist pens have a small window that allows you to see how much oil remains in the device. This feature is not available from all manufacturers. Not being able to visually estimate a device's fill level can make it difficult to know when a pen is empty. Once you feel there is no more oil in the non-Dosist device, simply throw it away.

Tips for How to Inhale

1. Relax! It's supposed to feel like a natural, deep breath.

2. Hold the battery with the attached oil cartridge at about 45 degrees, almost vertically, so the battery will heat the oil that is drawn into the bottom of the cartridge. If the cartridge is used while being held horizontally, it may not work properly.

3. Begin by inhaling two or three deep, slow breaths of air with your eyes closed before you start to use your vape. Feel the air going in and out of your lungs, and imagine you are trying to have your breath reach the very bottom of your lungs, almost touching your belly button.

4. When you are ready to take an inhalation, start with a slow inhale (air only) and right in the middle of the breath, inhale a 2-3 second puff of your vape followed by more clean air.

5. Exhale after about 3-5 seconds in a natural and relaxed motion.

6. The most common error patients make during inhalation is to close the throat so the vapor comes out of the nose and never actually arrives in the lungs. You can see if you are doing this by practicing in front of a mirror.

Oil Vapor Cartridges (Additional Battery Required)

When cannabis oil is vaporized using a cartridge, the extracted oil must be diluted so it can burn properly. There are several different types of oil vapor cartridge available on the market and all must be used with a separate battery. Below are the most popular cannabis oil cartridges available in cannabis dispensaries. All oil vapor cartridges contain diluents, discussed momentarily, which differ depending on the manufacturer.

CO_2 Oil Cartridges

Most vapor cartridges on the market today begin with a CO_2 extracted oil because, as previously mentioned, it is "solvent-free," resulting in a pure oil with no additives. The extracted oil is then mixed with ethanol to precipitate out the unwanted plant material. The final step in this production process is the evaporation of the ethanol. A benefit of a CO_2 vape cartridges is that they typically contain more of the naturally occurring plant cannabinoids and terpenes than a distillate oil that separates cannabinoids based on their boiling point. The final product for a CO_2 vape cartridge is an amber looking oil full of terpenes, and free of solvents, with approximately 50–70% potency. The higher the potency of the oil, the less you will need to use to reach your effective dose.

Distillate Oil Cartridges

Distillate oil is made through a process popular within the alcohol industry. In this case, boiling points are used to separate different components of the plant. The result is an extremely purified product containing isolated cannabinoids, such as THC, without the natural terpenes. Raw extracted cannabis oil is heated, and cannabinoids are collected while plant material such as chlorophyll and terpenes are removed. Terpenes are then added back into the final product to provide flavor and additional medicinal effects. Distillate oil is a highly purified cannabis oil with a potency of 80–90% and a very clean flavor.

Live Resin Oil Cartridges

Live resin oil, as a vapor cartridge, is not widely available. It is more frequently found as a concentrate but is becoming more and more popular in the cannabis industry for its full, robust flavor.

Live resin extraction is a process by which the freshly harvested flowers of the cannabis plant are flash-frozen and kept at temperatures below freezing while going through the extraction process. This is a time consuming and difficult process, which is why these products tend to be more expensive. But they are worth the effort and higher price. Live resin oil is extracted before drying and curing the flowers which retains all the natural terpenes within the plant for a final product bursting with flavor and medicinal value.

Diluents Used in Oil Vapor Cartridge: Know What's in Your Cartridge

Currently, the cannabis oil cartridge market in the United States is unregulated by the FDA. Therefore, additives and thinning agents used by some manufacturers are of inferior quality and need to be avoided at all costs. Patients *must* be aware of the diluents being used to make their preferred brand of vapor cartridges. This is not possible when purchasing from the black market.

Synthetic diluents, such as propylene glycol and polyethylene glycol, are inexpensive food additives that often cause throat and lung irritation when heated. Propylene glycol is one of the main ingredients in e-cigarette vape juice. Research has shown that noxious compounds such as formaldehyde and acetaldehyde can be formed when these diluents are heated and should, therefore, be avoided at all costs.

MCT, or micronized coconut oil, and vegetable glycerin are widely used as thinning agents in the cannabis vapor cartridge industry. There are no studies available regarding what happens when these products are heated and vaporized. Both products are considered food grade and are approved by the FDA for human consumption but not necessarily by means of vaporization. If these diluents irritate your lungs, I recommend you avoid them.

The optimal diluent for cannabis oil vapor cartridges is *cannabis*. In this case, the natural terpenes of the plant can be separated out and used to thin out thicker oils. Evolab, for instance, developed a unique CO_2 fractionation process to extract and purify a combination of cannabis terpenes (terpenoids and other phyto-chemicals) that is called Cannabis Derived Cutting Agent (CDCA). Some manufacturers say they use terpenes, but in reality, they are knockoff terpene products from cleaning agents that are sold in bulk. These are not high-quality, cannabis-derived terpenes. Look for products that use terpenes sourced from cannabis or plants only. Terpenes derived from fruits can create products with different flavors like mango and apple.

The bottom line when choosing a vapor cartridge is to look for a quality manufacturer that uses natural terpene thinning agents that do not feel harsh when inhaled. Look for cartridges labeled "Pure," meaning only cannabis products are used in the product. Never purchase a black market cartridge. If your vapor cartridge causes your throat to burn, chances are the cannabis oil is diluted using cheap, unsafe ingredients. As medical patients, we must hold manufacturers to the highest standards of safety and demand only pure, cannabis-containing products.

Vapor Cartridge Hardware Styles

Cartridges that hold and vaporize cannabis oil are available in several styles with subtle differences between products. Almost all cartridges today have a 510 thread that fits into most standard batteries on the market. The volume of a cartridge is typically 0.5ml or 1ml depending on the manufacturer, but can be as small as 0.3ml.

Cartridges heat and vaporize oil through one of two methods: the use of a cotton wick, or a metal or ceramic atomizer. Vapor cartridges with a cotton wick are falling out of favor because of a high failure rate. If you accidentally burn a cartridge with a cotton wick on a battery that is set at too high a temperature, you can easily ruin the taste of the oil or deactivate the cartridge completely. Deactivation of a cartridge happens when a battery is too hot. If you try to inhale from a deactivated cartridge, nothing will happen. I have seen many patients upset at the loss of an expensive cartridge full of oil that is no longer usable.

Several years ago, when I took my first trip to Colorado to visit some dispensaries and learn about products, I visited a very large, well-known dispensary to purchase some items for the weekend. I purchased two empty vapor cartridges with cotton wicks and some vape oil to fill them. Unfortunately, no one informed me that I needed to keep my battery temperature well below 4.0V, and I ended up burning out both cartridges very quickly (and lost the oil inside).

Vapor cartridges, such as CCELL, use a metal atomizer or a ceramic coil instead of a cotton wick to vaporize oil consistently and are less likely to burn the oil. Cartridges with atomizers have a lower failure rate and are better at retaining the flavor of your oil all the way to the last puff. If you taste a burnt taste when vaporizing your oil, it has been burned due to a hot battery and cannot be saved. Do yourself a favor and throw away the cartridge.

Pre-Filled Cartridges versus Fill-It-Yourself Cartridges

Cannabis oil cartridges are sold in medical and recreational dispensaries either already filled with oil or as a refillable, empty container. For beginners, I recommend a pre-filled oil cartridge (0.5ml or 1ml) that is ready to go when you take it out of the box. Place the cartridge on your battery, set it to the proper temperature, and inhale. When the oil is gone, you simply throw the empty cartridge away.

Alternately, cannabis vapor oil is sold in a "bulk", or multi-use container that is usually packaged in an oral syringe or small bottle that is poured into an empty vapor cartridge (sold separately). Thin oils like these tend to be heavily diluted, so be aware of what diluents are being used in the making of your oil. Bulk oils may offer cost savings, but I would not recommend this method for new patients. I find when patients are unfamiliar with how to handle a cartridge, they end up spilling the oil and wasting their product (sad moments).

Vapor cartridge components break down over time, and it can be difficult for patients to know when to discard refillable cartridges. Once the cartridge burns out, it is nearly impossible to extract the remaining oil in the cartridge. If new to vaporizing cannabis, keep it simple with a pre-filled, ready-to-go cartridge brand that uses cannabis terpenes as the diluent.

Everything You Need to Know About Batteries for Cartridges and Concentrates

The battery you choose to use with your vapor cartridge is one of the most important choices you will make when investing in equipment. The good news is, a high-quality battery is fairly inexpensive and can last for years.

If you decide that vaporizing cannabis oil is the delivery method that works for you, I highly recommend investing in a battery that is easy to use, has a long battery life, and will work consistently. There seems to be an unlimited number of batteries on the market today, but there are only five different *styles* of batteries made by multiple manufacturers. Most cartridges sold in dispensaries are designed to operate between 2.3V and 4.5V, so stay away from the super-powerful e-cig batteries.

When purchasing a vapor cartridge, be sure to ask about the proper operating temperature. If the dispensary employee is unsure (very possible because there are many products on the market), the rule of thumb is to start with lowest temperature setting on your battery and *slowly* increase the temperature until the oil flows easily. Thinner oils require lower temperatures, even 2.5V or below, and thicker oils may require a temperature of 3.0V–4.5V. Lower temperatures retain better flavor and prevent unnecessary harshness while inhaling, so err on the side of a lower temperature.

Cannabis cartridges are delicate and must be used on low temperatures to operate properly. Additional devices, such as a Yocan Cerum, can be attached to your battery for use with concentrates, but still do not require temperature above 5.0V. Excess heat and very high temperatures can irritate your throat and harm delicate lung tissue, so keep temperatures as low as possible.

If you are unable to get a good inhalation or feel like you are inhaling through a small straw, slowly increase the battery temperature until the oil is flowing freely. One long press of the battery button on a high temperature can ruin your cartridge (and your day). I can't count how many patients have burned their cartridges with the use of a high-temperature battery.

I bought my Eleaf Istick 20W mini **MOD (modified device) battery** several years ago for $30, and it's still going strong. It has a display for temperature and battery life, so I am never caught by surprise with a dead battery. A MOD battery is a box-like device that makes it easy to keep the cartridge upright, something which is necessary if it is going to function properly. This battery has a minimum temperature of 3V and may be too strong for very thin oils.

There are dozens of batteries sold for around $10, commonly marketed as **EVOD batteries**, and all I have to say is that you get what you pay for. These batteries have one to three temperature settings that you cycle through by hitting the button three times. The battery turns on and off by hitting the button five times fast, which can make it difficult for some people to operate. There are a million knockoffs that I have seen burn cartridges and literally fall apart. Look for a high-quality variable voltage battery such as the STR8 Revolve EVOD Vape Battery that allows you to adjust the temperature easily with a turn of the dial at the bottom of the unit. These are a bit more expensive, but worth the money.

For those patients who have dexterity issues and do not want to push a small button to activate their battery, CCell and O-Pen offer buttonless draw-activated batteries. After attaching the cartridge, patients simply inhale slowly and gently to turn on the device.

The Pax Era and the CCell Dart don't use cartridges at all. Instead, they use pre-filled "pods" that attach easily to their own battery and activate when the user inhales. Both devices fit discreetly in the palm of your hand, have no buttons, and, besides having cool features, couldn't be any easier to use. **Pod vaporizers** are a fantastic medical device concept and can easily be used by patients with severe disabilities.

Quick Tips to Get the Most Out of Your Battery

1. Unplug your battery immediately after it reaches a full charge. Sitting on a charger can damage the battery.
2. Do a quick check of your temperature setting before inhaling. Just one inhale on a hot battery can discharge or ruin your cartridge.
3. If possible, have a charged backup battery. It's always a good idea to have a backup in case one fails.
4. Keep the temperature at or below 2.0V if you are not sure what temperature to start using.
5. If the cartridge does not produce a vapor, slowly increase the temperature of the battery until you achieve a solid inhale.
6. Occasionally, clean the connection on the battery (where the cartridge screws in). Oil can leak onto the battery where the cartridge connects, and it needs to be cleaned with a cotton swab and a little rubbing alcohol so the device will continue to operate properly.

Practice using your new device before you need it, but don't practice too much because it's easy to consume more medicine than you intended. And remember, if you cough or feel a burn in your throat, make sure your battery is on a low temperature setting, take smaller puffs and be sure your product does not contain dangerous diluents. If unable to discern what is being used in the oil vapor cartridges sold in your dispensary, consider using a flower vaporizer.

CHAPTER 5

Sublingual Dosing

"Ending prohibition and the war on marijuana would be to admit to a catastrophic and irrational mistake from the side of government officials upholding an embarrassing tradition ... Instead of educating the public about the real risks and benefits of marijuana, millions of users were victimized and patients deprived from a medicine that has been effectively in use of more than five thousand years."
Sebastian Marincolo, PhD[1]
Author and Philosopher

Sublingual medications are applied to the side of the cheek or under the tongue for quick absorption and a fast response delivered within minutes. For patients who have trouble inhaling properly, or prefer something more discreet than vaporization, sublingual products deliver reliable, predictable relief.

Tinctures and oils that are designed to be used sublingually can also be consumed as an edible, which can give you more bang for your buck when shopping at the dispensary. In this chapter, I discuss the most common sublingual products found in cannabis dispensaries and some of the problems patients may face when choosing a sublingual dosage form. Once again, if you place a product on top of your tongue instead of under your tongue, you run the risk of swallowing the dose and waiting at least an hour for it to begin working. So be sure to administer products correctly to get that fast response.

Sublingual Products Available in Dispensaries

In every pharmacy across the globe, you will find different liquid formulations labeled as solutions, suspensions (shake well), or tinctures. A solution is defined as a homogenous mixture of two or more substances (no shaking required) while a suspension needs to be shaken before being consumed. Apparently, cannabis manufacturers have an aversion to the word "solution", since most products I found throughout the cannabis industry that should be labeled as a solution are given the misnomer of tincture or elixir.

Oils

Pure, CO_2 extracted cannabis **oil** can be placed directly under the tongue for sublingual administration, but may not be the most pleasant product you have ever tried. Thick oils can be slow to absorb or can get all over your teeth, so look for products that have a thinner consistency. Patients using pure cannabis oil in a syringe may find it difficult to measure an accurate or small dose, therefore a solution or tincture may be a better option.

The best part of using a cannabis oil for sublingual administration is the lack of additional diluents. These products are pure and diluent free, perfect options for cannabis purists.

Tinctures

The pharmaceutical definition of a **tincture** is a solution that contains a drug dissolved in an alcohol base. Apparently, this rule does not apply to the recreational cannabis industry. Many, many products across the recreational market labeled as "tincture" do not contain a drop of alcohol. Medical cannabis programs are more consistent about using the proper naming system for their products, so if you are allergic to alcohol, be sure to check what base is being used for your cannabis tinctures.

Seven Cannabis tinctures, Dr. Raw tinctures, and Wink tinctures are sold throughout California and do not contain any alcohol. These products can be used sublingually, but may be better suited for oral administration. "Tinctures" in the cannabis market can contain vegetable glycerin, distilled coconut oil, MCT (micronized or fractionated coconut oil), or even peanut oil as the oil base of the product in place of alcohol. Always check inactive ingredients for possible allergens as well.

A true tincture is made by dissolving a drug in a high proof alcohol (traditionally, grain alcohol in pharmacies) and can be, shall we say, unpleasant to administer sublingually. (Gross is a more accurate assessment.) Applying alcohol under the tongue burns, which is the obvious reason why manufacturers choose other more palatable bases such as MCT. In fact, an alcohol-based tincture would be better administered as an edible than under the tongue simply for comfort.

Solutions

Solutions (mislabeled as a tincture) are ideal products for new cannabis users because patients can begin using them by measuring very small starting doses, as small as 1mg, and can easily increase the dose as needed to really "dial in" their dosage. Sublingual products should be administered to the cheek or under the tongue and allowed to absorb for 1–2 minutes. Do not eat or drink anything for about 10 minutes after administering. Again, tinctures and liquid solutions may best be administered as an edible, and are therefore ideal for diabetic patients because they do not contain the high sugar content found in most edible products.

How to Calculate Your Dose Using a Liquid Product

Labeling of liquid cannabis products is not uniform throughout the cannabis industry, which can lead to confusion between products. It is vital to know how many milligrams (mg) of each cannabinoid are contained in your entire product (total milliliters) and how many milligrams are contained in each dose.

Once you have this information, you can easily adjust your doses according to Chapter 3. Below is a simple formula to determine how many milligrams (mg) will be in each milliliter (ml) of your product.

How to Calculate Your Dose Using a Liquid Product

Divide total (mg) in bottle by the total (ml) in bottle = mg in 1 ml.

This is the milligrams in 1ml of your tincture. If a 1ml dose
is too high, then calculate the following:

0.5ml = mg in ml divided by 2

0.25ml = mg in ml divided by 4

"A drop" is not considered a real dose and cannot be extrapolated
to use in other products. Instead, focus on the use of milliliters (ml)
and milligrams (mg). Try to determine the number of milligrams (mg)
in your favorite dose in case you need to switch to a new product.
Knowing your dose in milligrams (mg) will make using a new product
much easier.

Elixirs

An **elixir** is defined as an aromatic solution of alcohol and water. Once
again, we run into the same issue in labeling as with "tinctures," a lack of
alcohol. Sow Eden Organics produces beautiful hemp solutions containing CBD oil combined with Primrose oil (and soy lecithin as an emulsi-
fier), yet they are marketed as an elixir. I think the word "elixir" sounds
more exotic than "solution," but it's still not an exact depiction of the
product.

Elixirs, like tinctures and solutions, can be used sublingually or swallowed to work like an edible. They can also be placed on the skin for
topical treatment of rashes, psoriasis, and burns. The oil used for the
base will determine how quickly the cannabinoids are absorbed into the
bloodstream. If you do not like the effects of one manufacturer, simply
try another with a different base.

Sprays

Sublingual cannabis sprays are one of the best ways to medicate private-ly and effectively. Sprays may not be widely available in the recreation-al market, but they are a very popular delivery system in the medical cannabis program in Connecticut. Absolute Extracts and Verra Wellness are two manufacturers that make sublingual sprays that are available in various recreational markets.

Sprays are produced by dissolving cannabinoids in a base of alco-hol or MCT oil, often with a little peppermint flavoring for fresh breath. Each spray will deliver 2.5mg or 5mg of THC and/or CBD depending on the manufacturer. Spray doses cannot be adjusted, so patients must have an appropriate tolerance.

I like sprays for senior patients who do not want to inhale their prod-ucts but need fast relief during the day. Patients who want to medicate with a spray will need to have adequate hand dexterity to push down on the pump mechanism. A small spray device may be difficult to ad-minister for people dealing with severe arthritis, Parkinson's disease, or multiple sclerosis. If you have trouble using your hands properly, ask to see the product to determine if you can administer it easily.

Sublingual Slips or Films

A **sublingual film slip** is a small strip of medicated film that dissolves under the tongue on contact. These products are similar in design to Listerine Breath Strips except they are placed under the tongue rather than on top of the tongue, and they do more than freshen your breath! Kin Slips are cannabis films offered in select California dispensaries and come in multiple strengths and flavors.

Slips, like sprays, require a bit of dexterity to administer, so they may not be appropriate for some patients. Film slips are extremely popular with patients in Connecticut, and I believe recreational manufactur-ers should be looking into making more of these discreet, popular, and fast-acting dosage products.

Marijuana: a Spanish slang
term which translates to
Mary + Jane.

CHAPTER 6

Edibles and Oral Products

"Marijuana ... results in far fewer deaths each year than swimming pool accidents. Government shouldn't make war on people over their personal, private and peaceful choices."
Lawrence Reed[1]
President of the Foundation for Economic Education

Edibles are a delicious, private way to medicate, but can easily create a lot of confusion for patients new to using cannabis as medicine. The long-acting effects of these oral formulations make them ideal for patients with chronic symptoms, but if you accidentally take too much, or misjudge the timing, you may find yourself feeling very uncomfortable for several hours.

Patients with access to edibles in recreational markets can choose from hundreds of delicious products including infused gummies, nut butters, chocolates, and breath mints that deliver between 2.5mg and 10mg of THC and/or CBD per dose, with higher strengths available in the medical dispensaries. Edibles that contain high amounts of sugar are not the best choice for people living with diabetes or a chronic inflammatory disease. For those patients, I recommend pills, capsules, or liquid solutions.

In this chapter, I'll discuss why edibles feel stronger than other products, the effect of combining alcohol with edibles, and some tips for calculating the prefect dose while making homemade edibles. (Dosing guidelines for THC, CBD, and CBN are in Chapter 3.)

Why Edibles Produce Stronger Psychotropic Effects Than Inhalation or Sublingual Dosing

A recent study out of Denver documents a review of cannabis-related emergency room visits and found more general visits were attributed to inhalation (avoid this by using 1 or 2 puffs only), but more acute psychiatric visits (hallucinations, panic attacks) were attributed to edibles.[2] The reason for the disparity is the process by which THC is metabolized when delivered by inhalation versus when consumed orally.

When cannabis is inhaled or administered sublingually, cannabinoids are administered directly to the bloodstream to begin working within minutes. Edibles, on the other hand, must first be broken down in the stomach and then absorbed through the small intestine before entering the liver where they undergo "first-pass metabolism" before continuing to circulate throughout the body. This process can take an hour or more.

The primary metabolite of THC (technically called Δ-9-THC) after first-pass metabolism is a molecule called 11-hydroxy-Δ-9-tetrahydrocannabinol (11-OH-THC). This molecule has stronger psychological properties than its predecessor, THC, and forms faster and in highest concentrations when THC is orally ingested.[3]

This means that a cannabis-infused cookie will produce stronger psychotropic effects than your vape at the same dose. This may be a possible explanation as to why many cannabis users prefer to inhale rather than eat their medicine, it simply provides for a more predictable and less psychotropic response. Studies show when THC is combined with CBD, it may slightly decrease the production of Δ-11-THC, thus increasing overall tolerability.[4] Ratios of 2:1 or higher CBD:THC can help significantly reduce THC euphoria, but medicating with edibles is still more likely to produce stronger psychotropic effects than when medicating by other methods.

The Effects of Combining Alcohol and THC Edibles

A recent study in *Clinical Chemistry* showed when cannabis was inhaled, concentrations of both THC (technically Δ-9-THC) and the psychoactive active metabolite Δ-11-THC were significantly higher when consumed with alcohol.[5] Although the study was only performed on nineteen participants, the results were clear: Your typical inhaled dose can feel *significantly* stronger and cause more impairment when consumed with just a few alcoholic drinks.

If you want to have a cocktail or two, avoid consuming cannabis within at least 4-6 hours before and after drinking.

Translating Cannabis Tincture as an Edible

Alcohol-based cannabis tinctures have been used in medicine as far back as the nineteenth century because they are relatively easy to produce, but the strong alcohol flavor can be difficult for patients to tolerate. To administer an alcohol-based tincture, dilute a measured dose in a small amount of milk or juice (about a shot glass) and swallow quickly. You can place the tincture in anything, really, just be sure to drink the entire volume of liquid containing the tincture in less than 5 minutes.

Vegetable glycerin can be used as an alternative to alcohol when making "tinctures" because of the sweet flavor, but it is not as potent as alcohol, has a more complicated extraction process, and the final product will not be as stable as an alcohol-based tincture. Still, vegetable glycerin offers a good alternative for children and patients unable to tolerate alcohol.

CBD and THC "Water Soluble" Nano-emulsions and Micro-emulsions

As you learned earlier, the cannabinoid containing trichomes of the cannabis plant form a sticky, oily substance called resin that is soluble in oil and alcohol. But, if cannabis is only soluble in oil or alcohol, what exactly are "water-soluble" products which are sold both over the counter and in dispensaries?

To make a CBD or THC molecule "water-soluble", is not truly accurate. A better description would be "water-friendly". By reducing the size of the oil droplets to a very small size, and combining them with a surfactant, the CBD or THC molecules become more dissolvable in water, as well as allowing for increased potency with higher blood levels (since our body is made mostly of water). This process produces a product called a **nano-emulsion. Micro-emulsions** follow the same process but do not shrink the oil droplets as much, and therefore requires you to use as much as ten times more surfactant to make the molecule "water-friendly". Large amounts of surfactants can lead to unpleasant side effects. So, stick with nano-emulsions if given the choice.

With a higher bioavailability than edibles, water-soluble emulsions require a lower dose and provide a faster onset than regular edibles and solutions. Nano-emulsions can be taken orally or applied to the skin.

Homemade Edibles

Exclusively using edibles to medicate can become oppressively expensive. In addition, most edibles on the market contain high amounts of sugar, which may exacerbate inflammation in the body and cause a worsening of symptoms. If you decide edibles are your favorite way to medicate, I would strongly encourage you to educate yourself about how to make your own cannabis-infused butters, tinctures, and other edibles. There are hundreds of videos on YouTube on how to make cannabis butter, but my favorites include Nonna Marijuana, a ninety-something-year-old grandmother who's has been cooking with cannabis for years (even though she does not consume it). Search for "Weed Grandma Shows Us How to 420 Braise It: BONG APPÉTIT" for a great chicken cacciatore recipe and a giggle. I make infused CBD coconut butter from cannabis flowers that contain 18% CBD with only 1% THC. The result is an oil which has about 25–30mg per half teaspoonful (my favorite dose), totaling over 5000mg for $200. For anyone who regularly uses CBD, this is a huge cost savings.

Cooking with cannabis is a skill almost anyone can learn. I highly recommend purchasing a cookbook like *The Official High Times Cannabis Cookbook* and practice making different butters and tinctures. Some will be a hit and others a miss, but once you learn how to cook with cannabis, you can make any edible you want: gummies, chocolates, and even cannabis-infused jalapeño maple bacon (best thing ever). Cannabinoids are absorbed into the body using additional fats, so make sure to have a little fat with each dose of your edible for maximum effect.

To make an infused cannabis butter, you must first decarboxylate the cannabinoids within the dried cannabis flower. If you want to make things foolproof, the Nova Decarboxylator is a little machine that can retain up to 20% more cannabinoids than when a home oven is used. Once the flower is decarboxylated, it can be placed in a Magical Butter Machine (requires a minimum of 2 cups of oil) where you literally set it and forget it. Once the buzzer goes off, strain out the flower and *voila!* you have fresh, infused cannabis oil butter or tincture. Cannabis butter/ oil can be consumed as a spread on a bit of food or used in place of traditional oil when baking or cooking. Cannabis edibles can be made in bulk, wrapped individually and kept in the freezer for up to six months.

Purchasing cannabis flowers in a dispensary provides all the information needed to calculate how many milligrams of THC (and CBD) will end up in your final butter or tincture. If you calculate the milligrams in each teaspoonful of butter, then you'll be able to calculate how many milligrams will be in each brownie. Knowing how much THC is in each edible will give you a much more predictable, and medical, response.

If you really want to see what a professional chef can do when cooking with cannabis, watch "Bong Appetite" on the Vice channel. It is truly inspiring.

Before you make your edibles, you'll need to figure out how many milligrams of THC or CBD are in your flower products.

How to Calculate Milligrams (mg) of THC or CBD in Cannabis Flower

Step 1: Choose your butter and cannabis flower. I like coconut oil, but any high fat oil is fine. For this example, we will use 14 grams of flower.

Step 2: Add together the percentage of THC and THCA on the container's label. Use this number for THC in the equation below.

How to Calculate Milligrams (mg) of THC or CBD in Cannabis Flower

(1000 x %THC from label) x grams of flower = amount of THC in your flower

Example: 14 grams of 18% THC flower is
1000 x 0.18=180mg THC x 14grams

This equals 2520 milligrams of THC total
(that's a lot of THC!).

If using the Magical Butter Machine, which requires a 2 cup minimum (96 teaspoons) of oil, each teaspoonful will have approximately 25mg of THC. A quarter of a teaspoon will have about 6mg, which means that you will have over 380 doses. If 14 grams of flower has an average price of $125, that works out to about thirty cents for each dose! Patients can medicate every 8 hours for under a dollar a day.

CHAPTER 7

Topical Applications for Cannabis Oil

*"The full potential of this remarkable substance, including its
full medical potential, will be realized only when we end that regime
of prohibition established two generations ago."*
Lester Grinspoon M.D.[1]
Author of *Marihuana: The Forbidden Medicine*

Cannabis oil is derived when bulky plant material is removed and cannabinoids are concentrated into a nutrient-dense oil, which can then be
applied to the skin. CO_2 extracted oil is antibacterial and antitumoral
and offers substantial pain relief when used on burns and wounds. Ca-
nadian Rick Simpson was among the first people to discover the benefits
of cannabis oil applied to the skin when he applied his Rick Simpson Oil
(RSO recipe available at phoenixtears.ca) to a basal cell carcinoma and
made history when it healed.

Most of the research regarding topical cannabis use is emerging
science because people simply experiment with cannabis oil after other
numerous prescription drugs have failed to resolve the issue. Endocannabinoid receptors are found on the skin, therefore treatment with cannabis
is likely to produce positive results for a myriad of dermatological issues.[2]

Jack

One of the strangest wounds I've seen in a dispensary (or anywhere else for that matter) was on a man named Jack who was

seventy years old and had an open, weeping wound on the side of his neck. It looked like a fairly fresh wound, but he told me the wound had been exactly the same for the last fifteen years as a result of excessive radiation administered for his throat cancer. Jack complained about how the wound itched incessantly and had to always be bandaged because it was constantly weeping fluid. He had tried every prescription cream available, to no avail.

I recommended applying a small amount (enough to cover the wound but not drench it) of undiluted cannabis oil from a 1ml syringe containing 250mg of both CBD and THC to his wound every night, and to cover it with an occlusive dressing like Tegaderm. The oil I recommended for Jack was thin and easy to manipulate so it would spread easily onto the wound. Some oils can be thick and difficult to maneuver. The dressing would prevent air from entering the wound and allow the oil to penetrate more deeply (and keep the sheets clean). I told him to wash the oil off with soap and water or rubbing alcohol every morning.

After about two weeks of using the oil every night, he came in for a refill. I noticed that his wound was practically healed. I was truly shocked at the dramatic change. He'd tried a CBD + THC lotion (a diluted oil) for the daytime itch but found the undiluted oils much more effective. He wound up using the CBD + THC lotion on his achy knees. This wonderful, kind man had been suffering for fifteen years with a weepy, messy, itchy wound and now had a safe, effective, and permanent solution. That's the power of the cannabis plant!

A study published in *Pediatric Dermatology* exemplifies what happens when people are willing to try cannabis oil on otherwise untreatable skin conditions. In this small study, patients took it upon themselves to apply CBD oil to painful, blistering lesions caused by a rare genetic condition called Epidermolysis Bullosa, and all three cases resulted in "faster wound healing, less blistering, and amelioration of pain with cannabidiol use."[3] One patient was able to completely stop using opioid pain medications with only the use of topical CBD oil. Now, if that is not considered miraculous results, I don't know what is.

Topical cannabinoid use has shown great promise when used for itching.[4] Patients with psoriasis, atopic dermatitis, or eczema that is resistant to topical corticosteroids can often find relief when they apply whole-plant cannabis oil.

In this chapter, I'll talk about two types of cannabis oil topical products—undiluted oil (full strength) and diluted oil (creams and lotions)—and the different ways to use them. A list of conditions where cannabis can be helpful is shown below. When delivering cannabinoids through the skin, THC does not cause the euphoria experienced with other delivery methods, so patients can apply it as often as needed.

Ways to Use Cannabis Oil on the Skin			
Burns	Psoriasis	Eczema	Tooth Pain
Warts	Cysts	Open Wounds	Joint Pain
Arthritis	Ulcers	Neuropathy	Phantom Limb Pain
Leg Cramps	Rosacea	Plantar Fasciitis	

Undiluted Cannabis Oils: CO_2 Extracted and RSO

In Connecticut and other states with medical cannabis programs, patients can purchase pure cannabis oil that is sold in *oral* syringes (no needles!). The oral syringe prevents air from degrading the cannabinoids and makes for a simpler way to determine a specific dosage.

These days, large manufacturers of cannabis oil do not use the RSO extraction technique. Instead, they use industrial size CO_2 extraction machines that produce a microbially sterile product that tends to be thinner and more malleable. A small syringe of cannabis oil will hold hundreds, if not thousands, of milligrams of THC and CBD.

Treating Wounds, Ulcers, and Skin Cancer

Some wounds just won't heal. Whether due to trauma or a patient's compromised immune system, people can live with painful open wounds, ulcers, or skin cancers for months to years. Open wounds allow the infection to enter the body and can be very dangerous. Undiluted cannabis oil is a full-strength, cannabinoid dense oil that can be applied to troublesome, painful wounds to help relieve pain and accelerate wound healing.[5]

The New York Department of Health reports that the two most common bacteria to cause skin infections are Group A Streptococcus (GAS) and Staphylococcus aureus. Both are gram-positive types of skin bacteria.[6] A 2018 study from the *Journal of Integrative Medicine* concluded that cannabis extracts have the potential for the control of both hospital and community acquired MRSA.[7] MRSA (*methicillin-resistant* Staphylococcus aureus) is one of the deadliest skin infections people face today. GAS is just as deadly. You may know it better by its common name: flesh-eating bacteria.[8]

Skin infections such as these can potentially be treated with cannabis oil placed directly on the wound to immediately reduce damage and treat pain, while also enhancing wound healing as intravenous antibiotics continue to work systemically. For patients dealing with these kinds of life-threatening infections, there is literally no other topical option available to them.

Cannabis oil used to treat wounds should ideally be tested for pesticides, bacteria, mold, and fungus. You do not want to cause a secondary infection by using an oil that contains bacteria or fungus. These oils, when produced properly, can reduce pain and accelerate healing in wounds that have been otherwise unable to heal.

When looking to treat a wound with cannabis oil, first, purchase a syringe of CO_2 extracted cannabis oil that contains at least 250mg THC per 1ml. In my opinion, the oil should be very strong, much like the oils produced by the Rick Simpson Oil (RSO) method (phoenixtears. ca). Heavily diluted oils may not be as effective at fighting infection and reducing pain.

Second, clean and dry the wound and the surrounding area well.

Third, apply enough cannabis oil to cover the wound and a small area surrounding it.

Fourth, cover with an occlusive dressing (Tegaderm) that will work to keep the air out and help the oil to penetrate deeply.

Lastly, leave on for 12–24 hours, clean the wound well and repeat until healed. Use alcohol or very soapy, warm water to clean the oil from surrounding tissues.

If you experience increased levels of pain or the wound seems to be getting worse, stop treatment immediately and consult your physician. Both THC and CBD should help to decrease pain, so if there is any increase in pain, the wound absolutely should be examined by your physician as soon as possible.

Treating Warts

A wart is a virus that protrudes from the skin and, sorry to say, has no cure. After treatment, the virus goes dormant in the body and can reappear again and again. Treatments for warts have not changed in the last half a century and include "burning" the wart with liquid nitrogen or applying a topical product containing salicylic acid for up to two months.

Not surprisingly, I was unable to find a single study where cannabinoids have been used to treat warts. As an athlete, I have picked up a wart or two from the dirty gyms I inhabit. I have always treated warts at home with liquid nitrogen, but this painful treatment usually leaves a scar.

After placing my face on a contaminated yoga mat at the gym, I wound up with a small wart on my cheek. I did not want to risk a scar from the liquid nitrogen nor did I want to wait weeks for a topical product to work, so I decided to try an old home remedy for warts, duct tape. But this time I added my own twist, THC cannabis oil.

Duct tape has been so popular and successful at treating warts that a study was published in *Archives of Pediatrics and Adolescent Medicine*.[9] It can take several weeks for the duct tape to work and the wart to

117

disappear, so I decided to apply a small amount of undiluted, THC cannabis oil to the wart at bedtime and cover it with a small piece of duct tape. Every morning, I removed the tape and washed off the oil. To my surprise, the wart was completely healed in under a week with no scarring, and it never came back.

I have continued to use this process again and again on my hands and feet, with continued success. It is safe, pain-free, and faster than any other treatment I have tried in my forty plus years of dealing with annoying warts.

Diluted Oils: Lotions and Creams

The most common diluted cannabis oil products in both recreational and medical dispensaries are creams, ointments, and lotions. CBD balms (sold over the counter) went mainstream when Sephora, one of the largest suppliers of beauty products in the world, started carrying several CBD lotions and serums and over a dozen hemp beauty products. When shopping at retailers that sell CBD products, look for items that specifically list the amount of CBD within the jar, and buy the strongest product you can find.

As a single molecule, CBD is excellent for both pain and inflammation, but the addition of THC will add significant medical benefits to any topical product. If you are unable to procure products with THC, look for the strongest over the counter CBD product you can find. CBD topicals can be used to treat psoriasis, eczema, pain, neuropathy, and inflammation due to arthritis. Refer to Chapter 2 for benefits available from CBD.

Products that include both THC and CBD can be used for just about anything and may be more effective for relieving pain than products that have CBD by itself. Apply these creams and lotions to painful knees and hands as often as needed. As a patient with access to cannabis dispensary products, you can purchase products that contain both THC and CBD, so take advantage and buy the strongest products available that contain as many cannabinoids as you can get. *But be aware, THC is absorbed into the bloodstream when applied topically and will show up on a drug test.*

If you cannot find a satisfactory topical product (or if they are over-priced), you can easily compound your own balms at home with a simple mix of coconut oil and cannabis oil. Because coconut oil melts at 76°F (24°C), it is hard to overheat and destroy your cannabinoids when using it as a base.

To make a simple balm, purchase 1 gram of an indica CO_2 extracted concentrated oil (no butane extractions) such as a shatter or wax and stir into 1/4-1/2 cup of melted coconut oil. If the cannabis oil does not incorporate fully into the heated coconut oil, place the mixture on the stove at the lowest possible temperature for a minute or two until the cannabis oil fully dissolves in the coconut oil. Do not heat cannabis oil above 240°F (115°C) or you risk inactivating your product and render-ing it worthless. Low and slow is always the way to go when it comes to cooking with cannabis!

CO_2 extracted concentrated cannabis oils (called concentrates, shat-ters, and waxes) are among the purest products available in the dispen-sary and will create a strong topical product that can be used for pain, inflammation (if it contains CBD), scrapes, and minor skin burns. The more cannabinoids in your final product the better.

Apply lotions and creams up to six times a day to the affected area until it feels better. Topical products are inexpensive and can last for months to years if stored in a cool, dark, and dry location.

Treating Burns

Burns to the skin are extremely painful and have a limited number of prescription and over the counter treatments. The most dangerous part of a burn is the exposure of the body to infection through the damaged skin. Lidocaine is available over the counter as a topical numbing agent in combination with a topical antibiotic, while more severe burns are treated with a prescription cream containing silver sulfadiazine. Cannabis oil contains antibacterial properties that can prevent and treat infection while soothing pain, which makes it an ideal candidate for treating painful burns.[10]

To treat a burn at home, including sunburn, apply a balm of cannabis oil that includes high concentrations of THC as soon as possible. Re-apply as needed, as much as every 15 minutes. As the wound heals, you will need to apply it less often. If the burn begins to blister and open, clean often with soap and water, dry, and continue to apply your cannabis oil.

For a more severe burn, the risk of infection increases. Make sure to clean the wound regularly and apply a more concentrated, undiluted cannabis oil if required. The pain from the burn should lessen substantially with time and healing will improve using the cannabis oil. If the burn seems to get worse or does not seem to be healing properly, make sure to have your doctor or dermatologist look at it as soon as possible.

What Are Patches All About

Transdermal patches are carried by a limited number of dispensaries and are a great option for a low dose delivery method that lasts for hours and does not have psychoactive or euphoric effects. Pure Ratio patches can deliver medication for up to 96 hours while Mary's Medicinals patches work within 15–30 minutes and last for 8–12 hours.

Transdermal patch delivery systems are the most complicated delivery system available, and their steep price reflects the extra work required in the manufacturing process. Each patch must deliver a slow, steady release of the drug into the bloodstream while avoiding "dumping" medication into the system from applied heat or if the patch is accidentally bumped.

Transdermal patches can be expensive but are a fantastic option for patients looking for long-acting relief for pain or sleep disturbances without the psychoactive side effects produced when inhaled or consumed as an edible. If you can find these patches in a dispensary, they tend to be for people with a low tolerance, which is perfect for new cannabis patients. Apply to clean, dry skin, and rotate the application site. Avoid using while in a jacuzzi or heated swimming pool.

SECTION 3

Diseases

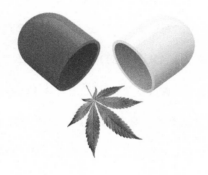

A recent study published in *The European Journal of Internal Medicine*, surveyed over 2,700 Israeli patients 65 years and older who received medical cannabis as a treatment for several conditions. More than 93% reported a drop in their pain levels.

CHAPTER 8

Pain Due to Injury, Neuropathic Pain, and Inflammation

"I have seen many patients with chronic pain, muscle spasms, nausea, anorexia, and other unpleasant symptoms obtain significant—often remarkable—relief from cannabis medicines, well beyond what had been provided by traditional (usually opiate-based) pain relievers."
David Hadorn, MD, PHD[1]
Medical Consultant for GW Pharmaceuticals, LTD

Chronic pain impacts over 20% of our nation's population. That's almost *seventy million* adults in the United States who live with the emotional stress and physical restrictions of unremitting pain.[2] The psychological effects of living with chronic pain can be just as debilitating as the pain itself. Patients who live with pain can find getting a restful night's sleep nearly impossible. Incessant pain coupled with a lack of sleep leads to irritability, depression, and anxiety that inevitably leads to broken marriages, lost friends, and a lack of joy for living.

Classification of Pain

The Johns Hopkins Blaustein Pain Treatment Center treats twenty-seven different causes of pain, all of which can be treated with cannabis.[3] For the purpose of this book, we will focus on three main categories of pain and how to effectively use cannabis to treat them:

Nociceptive Pain—pain due to injury or physical damage

Neuropathic Pain—nerve pain

Inflammation—activation of the inflammatory process (rheumatoid arthritis, psoriatic arthritis) causing acute/localized or systemic/chronic inflammation that leads to pain

In reality, pain classifications tend to overlap, and patients often experience all three types of pain at once, which is best treated with multiple cannabinoids. In this chapter, I'll talk about the current pharmaceutical interventions for nociceptive pain, nerve pain, and inflammation and how suitable cannabis products can help you reduce or even eliminate the dangerous prescription medications (including opioids, anti-inflammatory pills, muscle relaxants and neuropathy treatments) you might be using.

Nociceptive Pain Treatments (Pain from Injury)

The Merck Manual of Diagnosis and Therapy says that nociceptive pain, the most common type of pain, is a result of stimulation of pain receptors from tissue injury, which are located in the skin and internal organs.[4] This type of pain will occur after surgery, a car accident, a sprain, or damage to internal organs. Nociceptive pain is described as sharp or dull, aching, and throbbing, and it may be constant or intermittent. As cancer invades bones and organs, most of the pain generated is nociceptive type pain.

Why Opioids for Pain Relief

Opium, derived from the opium poppy, has been used in medicine, like cannabis, for thousands of years. The most widely accepted pharmaceutical treatment for nociceptive pain is the use of opioids, which originated with morphine from the opium poppy. "Opioids have been regarded for millennia as among the most effective drugs for the treatment of pain. Their use in the management of acute severe pain and chronic pain related to advanced medical illness is considered the standard of care in most of the world."[5]

126

Opioid use for chronic pain exploded in the mid-1990s with expanded prescribing of long-acting, high dose opioids for everything from knee pain to acute post-surgery pain. The result of this massive over prescribing of opioids has spawned generations of addicted patients.

Addiction is a two-prong process. First, the substance involved must induce a significant withdrawal response once removed. Many things, like caffeine and sugar, can cause withdrawal, but they don't necessarily ruin lives as opioids can. This brings us to the second, and more insidious, aspect of addiction—extreme negative changes in behavior (intense drug craving and compulsive use). The opioid receptor system influences both areas of addiction, pain and behavior, which may explain why opioid addiction is so deeply destructive.

Our body contains three main opioid receptors, mu-, delta-, and kappa-opioid receptors. **The opioid receptor system** is responsible for pain modulation *and* addiction, which is why it is responsible for both decreasing pain *and* causing addictive behavior.[6] Our opioid receptor system also influences "emotional response, epileptic seizures, immune function, feeding, obesity, respiratory and cardiovascular control as well as some neurodegenerative disorders."[7] This glaring issue of brutal and deadly addiction may be able to be avoided in a large number of patients when using cannabis to treat pain since the withdrawal from cannabis was equated to caffeine withdrawal in a government-funded, 1994 NIDA study.[8] Some patients may experience more intense withdrawal symptoms from cannabis than others, but no one is destroying their life for another cup of coffee.

Another important aspect of the opioid receptor system is the existence of receptors in the lungs and areas of the brain responsible for the respiratory functions of the body. When high doses of opioids are consumed or mixed with other depressants (alcohol and benzodiazepines for example), patients increase their risk of decreased respiration resulting in death. This deadly side effect is being played out across the United States where hundreds of thousands of people have lost their lives due to opioid toxicity.[9] This issue does not exist when pain is treated with cannabis since endocannabinoid receptors are not contained in the lungs or parts of the brain responsible for respiratory functions (medulla oblongata), and therefore do not produce respiratory depression when consumed in excess.[10] Patients should still use great care when combining opioids with cannabis as other negative side effects, such as increased sedation, can occur.

Finally, opioids have been linked to the worsening of dementia and, therefore, should be avoided in older patients, the exact group of people most likely to have increased levels of chronic pain.[11]

Cannabis for Nociceptive Pain Relief

An online survey of 1,321 subjects published in *The Journal of Pain* reports that more than 80% of the participants "reported substituting cannabis for traditional pain medications (53% for opioids, 22% for benzodiazepines), citing fewer side effects and better symptom management as their rationale for doing so."[12] I have witnessed hundreds of patients replace their opioid medications with cannabis when treating both acute and chronic pain without experiencing the kinds of withdrawal effects normally seen with chronic opioid use.

One patient I met with, Ken, was able to stop taking his opioid medication less than 36 hours after completion of major shoulder surgery by substituting them with an oral 2:1 CBD:THC tincture. His anesthesiologist was fascinated by how he was able to completely stop his opioid use so soon after surgery, and by doing so felt more alert, relieved his opioid-related constipation, and he healed faster than expected.

In my experience, patients currently using medications such as tramadol or low dose hydrocodone (Vicodin) to treat their **moderate, chronic pain** may be able to substitute these medications with CBD-isolated products that do not contain additional THC. Patients can begin with 10-20mg of CBD and follow the guidelines in Chapter 3 regarding how to increase their dose to an effective level. If you reach doses of 50–75mg CBD with little relief, THC may need to be added for increased pain management.

Some patients who have been taking pain medication for an extended period of time are worried about stopping their pain pills in order to switch over to cannabis. This is a valid concern. First, you do not have to stop taking your pain pills upon starting cannabis therapy. Continue to take your pain medication as prescribed while you learn how to use cannabis effectively before you consider stopping the medication. The combination of THC with other sedating medications can cause you to feel extra sleepy, so be sure to keep your initial THC dosages low and decrease your opioid consumption as soon as you feel comfortable. Once you find the right dose and combination of cannabinoids, you will find you won't need to reach for your next pain pill after four hours. This is when you know you are on the right track.

Inform your pain management prescriber of your intent to decrease your opioid usage with the use of cannabis. When you are ready to reduce your use of pain medications, begin by first decreasing the amount of short-acting, or breakthrough, pain medication you use every day. If you are only taking a short-acting pain medication for pain management, then begin by decreasing one pill every 1 to 2 days. Once you no longer need your daily, short-acting opioids, you can completely switch over to cannabis for your daily pain needs and only use your opioids on days with increased levels of pain.

For others, removal of the short-acting opioid will leave you with a long-acting opioid as your primary source of pain management. Once the breakthrough pills are no longer needed, you can have your physician decrease the strength of your long-acting opioid over the next several weeks to months. As the strength of the long-acting opioid is decreased, you may need to increase your intake of CBD and THC to compensate. It should be a slow, natural progression that is done in conjunction with your doctor's advice, and you should not feel stressed, overly sedated, or feel increased levels of pain at any time during the process. As the opioids are removed, they should be seamlessly replaced by an adequate dosage of CBD and/or THC. Some patients may have pain that still requires daily opioids, but the dosages should be much lower when combined with cannabis.

For patients with **severe pain**, or if CBD is simply not strong enough, THC offers synergistic pain relief when combined with CBD. Based on my own observations, the ratio with the most success for pain relief is 1.7:1 CBD:THC. Chances are, you will not be able to find this exact product in most dispensaries, but a ratio of 2:1 or 3:1 CBD:THC offers excellent pain relief while having the added benefit of more tolerable psychoactive side effects. That's not to say you won't feel the effects of THC, but they will be a bit more mild.

Patients suffering from chronic, daily pain cannot and should not suddenly stop taking their pain medications throughout the day. In fact, without pain medication, these patients would not be able to work or function in life due to extreme physical pain. Therefore, reducing euphoric effects while treating pain with THC is necessary for patients who require around the clock pain medication.

If you find a 2:1 CBD:THC ratio too strong, try a 3:1, 4:1 or 5:1 CBD:THC product. The ratio needed is up to you. By consistently consuming the same dose of THC around the clock, most people find the side effects from THC become more tolerable. It is important to treat your pain effectively. It is always harder to overcome pain than it is to prevent it, so smaller doses around the clock are more comfortable and effective than large doses taken sporadically.

Using cannabis to treat pain offers a patient the ability to not have to continually increase their opioid dosage. Patients who consume opioids around the clock for relief of chronic pain will find that, over time, they need more and more medication to achieve the same level of pain relief.

This is intrinsic to opioids and is not due to patient behavior. By supplementing with cannabis, patients can reduce their overall opioid consumption and, therefore, will not require steady increases in dosages as with the sole use of opioids. In other words, the opioids will offer more pain relief when used less often than when dosed chronically at high doses.

At appropriate dosages, daytime formulations of the sativa variety offer excellent pain relief without extreme drowsiness, while indica varieties may offer better muscle relaxation. For daytime pain start with sativa-based products that include both CBD and THC. If ineffective for pain control, a hybrid or indica strain may offer better relaxation and, therefore, better relief, so plan on experimenting with different strains as well as different combinations of cannabinoids. Finding the perfect strain for your pain can take a little experimentation and patience, but with a better safety profile than opioids, medicating with cannabis puts the control back into your hands.

Neuropathic Treatments for Nerve Pain

Neuropathic pain is the result of damage to nerve fibers somewhere along the nervous system. Three common conditions associated with acute and chronic neuropathic pain are diabetic peripheral neuropathy (in hands and feet), painful post-herpetic neuralgia (shingles), and cancer. Sciatic type nerve pain is a common complaint in older adults and is often the result of worsening of a back injury, such as herniated or "bulging" discs. Neuropathy is experienced as pins and needles, burning, numbness, tingling, and shooting sensations that remain localized or radiate around the body and can result in a complete lack of feeling or numbness.

Neuropathy resulting from diabetes is a result of excess blood glucose damaging delicate nerve fibers in extremities. An injury to the spine can result in pain that radiates down one or both legs leading to numbness of the feet. Nerve damage is a common side effect of both chemotherapy and radiation, and pain can continue years after treatment has ended.

Pharmaceutical Treatments for Nerve Pain

Currently, there is no published data regarding to the prevalence of nerve pain in the United States. This is surprising considering the number of conditions associated with neuropathy as a listed side effect (radiation, herniated discs, diabetes). The most commonly used medications to treat neuropathy are non-steroidal anti-inflammatory drugs (NSAIDs), anti-depressants, opioids, and anti-epileptics drugs. As you can see, none of these medications specifically target nerve pain, which may explain their limited success.

The three most frequently prescribed medications for nerve pain are gabapentin, pregabalin (Lyrica), and duloxetine (Cymbalta), a se-rotonin and norepinephrine re-uptake inhibitor (SNRI) antidepressant. Each of these medications should not be stopped suddenly because of an increased risk of seizure. The most common side effects of all these drugs are sedation, fatigue, weight gain, and abnormal thinking. Dulox-etine (Cymbalta) carries an additional black box warning showing an increased risk of depression and suicide in some patients.

Black box warnings are required by the FDA on a certain prescrip-tion drug's label that have specific dangers associated with the drug. They are designed to call attention to serious or life-threatening risks.[13]

Cannabis Treatments for Nerve Pain

Cannabinoids mediate their effects through activation of endocannabi-noid receptors to decrease inflammation leading to nerve pain, either topically or systemically. The best products for treating nerve pain are rich in CBD and have low levels of THC (moderate to high THC may be required for more severe pain.) I have witnessed many people who were able to achieve considerable success when treating their nerve pain with isolated oral CBD products (tinctures, drops, and pills) containing little to no THC when gabapentin and pregabalin (Lyrica) failed to offer substantial relief or the side effects were intolerable.

Patients should begin treatment with CBD-isolated products and increase their dose as recommended in Chapter 3. Once a substantial dose of CBD is established (25–75mg per dose), patients who need more relief should consider slowly adding small amounts of THC (2–5mg) until pain subsides or side effects become overwhelming. (Sativa seems to work best for daytime nerve pain if tolerated.)

Moderate to severe nerve pain should be treated by sublingual or oral delivery because delivery by inhalation may make it difficult to find an effective dose of CBD, the main component needed to treat neuropathy.

If moderate levels of CBD with low levels of THC (for example, 25mg CBD with 5mg THC) are inadequate, the final step when treating severe nerve pain is high dose CBD (50–75mg per dose) with moderate to high doses of THC (as tolerated). These products are the strongest options available for treating neuropathy but also produce the most euphoria, so they may not be appropriate for some patients during working hours.

If nerve damage is localized, such as in the hands and feet, patients can begin treatment by applying topical CBD (added THC may help) to the area every few hours. Lotions and creams offer moderate pain relief for localized nerve pain and do not have systemic side effects. They can be combined with more powerful oral products for additional alleviation of pain.

Anti-Inflammatory Treatments

Acute inflammation occurs when the immune system sends fluid and white blood cells to an injury site to induce healing. Inflammation creates pain and swelling, which is most commonly treated with corticosteroids (prednisone), non-steroidal anti-inflammatories (naproxen, ibuprofen), and COX-2 inhibitors (Celebrex, Mobic). All of these drugs are effective when treating mild to moderate pain and inflammation but carry their own risks, especially with long-term use.

Patients treating acute inflammation should always limit their use of anti-inflammatory medications as much as possible. This becomes complicated when treating chronic conditions such as arthritis and multiple sclerosis, which require the use of anti-inflammatory medications for months to years. Long-term use of anti-inflammatory drugs can lead to stomach ulcerations, cardiac damage, and kidney dysfunction.

The problems associated with anti-inflammatory pharmaceutical medications do not cross over when using CBD, a potent anti-inflammatory molecule in its own right. When treating acute episodes of inflammation, CBD can be used alone or combined with NSAIDs like ibuprofen for short term use, increased pain relief and faster healing. Dosages of 25–75mg CBD can be taken every 6–8 hours for around the clock relief. Adding CBD to traditional pharmaceutical therapies can help treat pain more effectively while allowing for reduced dosages of the anti-inflammatory medications over time.

Chronic inflammation does not follow the same physiological pathway as acute inflammation and has been identified as among the most significant contributing factors to the development of chronic disease, such as multiple sclerosis and dementia. Chronic inflammation is described as a systemic, low-grade inflammation that can be measured by several inflammatory biomarkers. For instance, high levels of C-reactive protein have been linked to an increased risk of heart disease. High levels of Substance P, a pain transmitter, are seen in the spinal fluid of patients with fibromyalgia.[14]

A 2009 study in *Rejuvenation Research* showed how systemic inflammation influences pathophysiologic processes and contributes to chronic disease, frailty, disability, and mortality.[15] Currently, we do not have a single prescription medication that decreases underlying systemic inflammation. In fact, some of the most effective treatments for reducing chronic inflammation do not involve drugs at all.

Diet and lifestyle are two factors thought to contribute significantly to chronic inflammation and can be adjusted accordingly to reduce symptoms of disease. Turmeric, a spice widely used in Indian cuisine, has potent anti-inflammatory properties and may be beneficial for preventing and treating pain, Alzheimer's disease, heart disease, and cancer.

The first step when treating any chronic inflammatory issue is to remove processed foods and commit to a whole-food, plant-based diet. These types of dietary changes to promote healing are endorsed by The

Physicians Committee for Responsible Medicine (pcrm.org). Intermittent fasting has also been linked to improved biomarkers of disease, reduced oxidative stress, and improved insulin sensitivity.[16]

CBD (cannabidiol) is a potent antioxidant and anti-inflammatory molecule that inhibits the expression of inflammatory cytokines and limits the harmful effects of an overactive inflammatory response leading to chronic inflammation.[17] It may be possible to use CBD to treat brain fog, nerve pain, and other issues related to systemic inflammation not treatable by current pharmaceuticals, and CBD has a better and safer side effect profile. When we decrease systemic inflammation using scheduled doses of CBD, almost like a supplement rather than a drug, we may be able to slow or resolve the progression of chronic disease symptoms. It may seem like a stretch, but based on all we know, CBD has that much medical potential. Only time, coupled with quality clinical studies, will determine how we can effectively use CBD to decrease the prevalence of chronic, systemic inflammatory disease.

Fibromyalgia

Fibromyalgia is an amplification of the body's pain response and an example of a chronic inflammatory disease. Diagnosing fibromyalgia is complicated, and its cause is unknown. Three independent studies showed fibromyalgia patients have unusually high levels of Substance P, a chemical in spinal fluid that helps transmit pain signals to the brain.[18, 19, 20]

The first scientific study of fibromyalgia confirmed the existence of symptoms and tender points in the body as far back as 1981, yet it was not until 2005 that the American Pain Society established guidelines for treating fibromyalgia and not until 2007 that the FDA approved the first drug for treating fibromyalgia (Lyrica).[21] It's interesting to note that more than 3/4 of fibromyalgia patients are women.[22]

The Mayo Clinic's website states that a fibromyalgia diagnosis can be made if a person has had widespread pain with no underlying medical condition for more than three months.[23] Other common symptoms are:

- tenderness to touch or pressure affecting muscles and sometimes joints or even the skin
- severe fatigue
- sleep problems (waking up unrefreshed)
- problems with memory or foggy thinking

Pharmacology approaches treatment using SNRI antidepressants (Cymbalta and Savella) or pregabalin (Lyrica), a drug with additional indications for neuropathy and seizures disorders. Duloxetine (Cymbalta) and milnacipran (Savella) increase levels of norepinephrine and serotonin in the brain but also contain FDA black box warnings for an increased risk of suicide. Pregabalin (Lyrica) was the first drug specifically approved for fibromyalgia and has been shown to decrease nerve pain, although patients complain that lower doses may only be moderately effective, while higher dosages produce excessive sedation and weight gain.

It is highly probable that an imbalance within the endocannabinoid system is a significant contributing factor to the symptoms of fibromyalgia. Many patients with fibromyalgia also experience overlapping conditions such as irritable bowel syndrome, lupus, and arthritis. Whatever its cause, fibromyalgia is a total disruption of the body's homeostasis.

I have found cannabis to be overwhelmingly effective at reducing symptoms associated with fibromyalgia. Products high in CBD with low to moderate THC levels are effective when treating pain, insomnia (indica), depression (sativa), and fatigue (sativa) and can significantly improve a patient's quality of life. Strains high in CBN may be useful for pain, inflammation and relaxation.

Complex Regional Pain Syndrome (CRPS)

CRPS is a chronic, expansive pain condition. Sufferers of CRPS experience a pain response that is out of proportion to the associated injury.

CRPS often involves an injury to the arm or leg that "spreads" to other areas of the body. Another way to describe CRPS is as a massive malfunction of the nervous system.

As a pharmacist, I had not heard much about CRPS during my years in pharmacy but learned more about it as I consulted with patients in the dispensary. I find it to be one of the scariest and most frustrating conditions affecting patients because there is no satisfactory answer regarding its cause or how it can be effectively treated. My first inclination is to recommend acupuncture over drugs, but for many who suffer, medication is required.

One patient with CRPS had a surgical repair to her shoulder during which her surgeon accidentally damaged a nerve. The damaged nerve did not cause pain in her shoulder, rather her thumb and pointer finger appeared as if they were dipped in acid: The skin turned red and peeled off and the nails turned black. This woman lived with such extreme pain that she could not tolerate a bedsheet touching her fingers. Even topical cannabis creams, which I thought would offer at least some relief, were too strong to put on her damaged fingers, so she exclusively used inhaled and oral products.

One of the most severe cases of CRPS I observed was in a patient named Sam.

Sam

Sam arrived at his first cannabis consultation in a wheelchair pushed by his wife, Linda. He was eighty years old at the time, had previously led a very active lifestyle, and was desperate to decrease his current medication regimen, which was limiting his quality of life.

He told me that eighteen months earlier he'd had an aneurysm on his lower spine that had burst. He lost the use of his legs for about nine months and after much physical therapy was barely able to walk with a cane. The pain had progressed to the point where he was in excruciating pain from his knees to his feet 24 hours a day. His medication list was impressive: Kadian, 160mg twice a day (long-acting morphine); oxycodone 30mg every 4 hours if needed for breakthrough pain (and he needed it); baclofen; gabapentin; and on and on. The list contained about fifteen different medications for treating pain, inflammation, and muscle spasms. He and his insurance company were spending thousands and thousands of dollars on prescriptions every month, yet he was still living with terrible pain.

His pain management doctor was very creative and knowledgeable, but Sam was still oscillating between horrible pain and medicine-induced inebriation. He described how he would take half of a tablet oxycodone every 2 hours to prevent the pain, but sometimes he became so groggy that he relied on people around him to help him walk. His life had become unbearable; he needed help.

I showed Sam which prescriptions on his list he would be able to decrease (under the supervision of his physician) once he learned how to use cannabis and found a regimen that worked for him. He had never "smoked pot" before, so we decided to start him on a high CBD, low THC oral regimen to help decrease the psychotropic side effects of the THC. Over time, his cannabis regimen became 40mg of CBD taken every 6–8 hours along with 10–20mg of THC taken every 8 hours. He never took more than 20mg of THC at once because more than that made him too drowsy. Sometimes Sam would take an extra CBD dose during the day if he felt he needed it.

Once he was comfortable with how to dose and adjust his cannabis products (which took about 2 weeks), his physician began to lower his morphine (Kadian), baclofen, gabapentin, and oxycodone doses. Every time he arrived at the dispensary for a refill he would, with a cane but independently, walk into the dispensary. After his first visit, I never saw him arrive in a wheelchair again.

More and more research studies support the use of cannabis as a viable treatment for pain. Cannabis is an excellent choice for people who cannot tolerate pharmaceutical options or simply find them ineffective. The freedom that comes with determining your specific combination of cannabinoids is not achievable with pharmaceutical therapies. Patients anchored to opioids or nerve pain medications are unable to suddenly stop their pills without risking serious, life-threatening complications. These issues may be able to be avoided when cannabis is used as the primary pain management medication.

Pot: a shortening of the
Spanish word "potiguaya";
a wine in which marijuana
buds are steeped.

CHAPTER 9

How to Begin Using Cannabis to Treat the Side Effects of Chemotherapy

*"We know that prohibition laws did nothing but waste money,
waste lives and destroy opportunities. It is not working.
And marijuana has been the engine driving the drug war."*
Joycelyn Elders, MD[1]
Former US Surgeon General

Cancer is described as "a battle," conceivably the biggest fight of one's life, so it is appropriate that the first drug discovered to help combat cancer, nitrogen mustard, was literally a drug of war. Soldiers exposed to mustard gas during World War II were found to have toxic changes in bone marrow cells that eventually led to the discovery of using these agents for treating lymphoma.[2]

During and after treatment with chemotherapy, patients can experience a long list of physical and emotional side effects that can last for years after treatment has ended and the cancer has gone into remission. Cannabis has a long history of use for pain, nausea, and to increase the appetite during cancer treatment, but more and more studies reveal the immense benefits cannabis can have on the body as a whole through neutralization of systemic inflammation and oxidative stress, as well as acting as a protective agent for internal organs from toxic chemotherapies that work to kill cancer cells.

In this chapter, I will show you how cannabis may be used to actually prevent damage to the body from toxic chemotherapeutic agents, as well as being used to combat some of the most common side effects of chemo-therapy and radiation, such as those listed by the American Cancer Society:

- fatigue
- depression (mood changes)
- appetite changes and excessive weight loss
- pain
- inflammation
- nausea and vomiting
- infection
- skin changes

Pharmaceutical Treatments for Chemotherapy Side Effects

As therapies to treat cancer continue to advance every year, supportive care to combat chemotherapy side effects has remained stagnant. As treatments drag on, reactions to chemo-toxic agents require a plethora of drugs to help patients endure and maintain a good quality of life.

Antacids, steroids, pills for nausea, antihistamines, antidepressants, pain medications, anti-anxiety medications, more pain medications, pills to help stimulate the appetite, and the list goes on. This creates a long, dizzying array of drugs with an even longer list of side effects and possible drug interactions that can leave patients feeling exhausted and dejected.

For most, the words "you have cancer" brings an immense amount of fear and anxiety. As treatment wages on, the fear for some can become almost overwhelming. Standard treatment includes a benzodiaz-epine (Xanax, Ativan or Valium) for anxiety and an antidepressant, as discussed in detail in Chapter 16. Antidepressants are limited in their effectiveness, take four to six weeks to begin working, and cause difficult withdrawal issues once patients decide they no longer wish to continue treatment, but are currently the only drug options available for patients.

After cancer treatment begins, many patients must endure bouts of nausea and vomiting that will be treated with a class of drugs called serotonin 5-HT3 receptor antagonists [ondansetron (Zofran) and granisetron (Kytril)]. These medications have drug interactions with most antidepressants (a substantial problem) and include common side effects of constipation and drowsiness, which can make an exhausted and fatigued patient feel even worse. A second powerful class of anti-nausea drugs, the P/neurokinin 1 (NK1) receptor antagonists, block the chemicals in the body that trigger nausea and vomiting. They contain a substantial list of drug interactions but actually hurt the wallet more than anything since they are priced at around $35 per pill.

Medications to increase appetite are essentially nonexistent. It is of vital importance that patients undergoing treatment for cancer do not lose excessive amounts of weight or they risk becoming too weak to continue treatment. Megestrol acetate (Megace) and the synthetic THC pill (dronabinol) are the only options currently available to help patients maintain an appetite, and neither option has shown to be particularly successful.

Pain is a common complaint of cancer patients who can quickly find themselves requiring higher and higher dosages of dangerous opioid medications from either the growth of the cancer or the chemotherapeutic agents being used to treat it. Opioid drugs come with their own intrinsic dangers and should not be combined with benzodiazepines used for anxiety because of the dangers of decreased respiration and death. For a substantial number of people, opioids can actually make anxiety worse.

Opioids cause increased drowsiness, fatigue, constipation, and exacerbate depressive symptoms, but are still currently the only option for pain that is covered by insurance and considered a first-line therapy for all patients. So, when the pain gets out of control and opioids are not working or are not well tolerated, where is a patient supposed to turn?

Gail

Gail was a Stage 4 lung cancer patient whose opioid use had escalated dramatically in the last several months and had become an increasing concern to herself, her husband and her oncologist. When I met Gail, she was taking 60mg of OxyContin every 8 hours plus 10mg oxycodone for breakthrough pain every 4 hours, but her pain continued to increase every week. With few options remaining, her oncologist recommended trying cannabis, although neither she, nor her husband believed it would actually work. By the time they arrived at the dispensary, Gail and her husband were desperate to try anything.

Gail was not interested in trying multiple products. She wanted one product that I believed would help reduce her pain and help her decrease her opioid use. I recommended a 2:1 CBD:THC (indica strain) tincture that was regularly available at the dispensary, so she would not have to deal with out of stock issues. It was an alcohol-based tincture that didn't taste very good, but I helped her find a way to take each dose comfortably. I gave Gail a dosing chart that helped her and her husband easily understand how to slowly increase the dose of the product over several days until she felt her pain subside.

They asked me how quickly it would be before Gail would be able to decrease her OxyContin dosage. I told them I believed that within three to five days of using the tincture Gail would no longer need to take her breakthrough oxycodone medication. I advised that once Gail did not need her breakthrough oxycodone, she should ask her oncologist about reducing the OxyContin dosage. After about three weeks, Gail had decreased her OxyContin dosage from 60mg to 10mg every 8 hours and no longer needed any medication for breakthrough pain.

Cannabis Treatments for the Side Effects of Chemotherapy

Cannabis can treat several conditions related to chemotherapy simultaneously, thus reducing the need for multiple medications that include the potential for drug interactions, have multiple side effects, and can be cost-prohibitive. Most oncology nurses can tell you that for decades cannabis has been the best-kept secret on any oncology ward. People who use cannabis to combat symptoms during treatment can find relief for fatigue, depression, pain, and nausea with the use of a single sativa product, something totally unheard of when using today's pharmacology options. Also, patients can taper the treatment to their tolerance, thus returning a small sense of control to themselves, something many patients feel is lost when presented with a cancer diagnosis.

Fatigue and Depression

The uplifting terpenes of a sativa strain can help combat both fatigue and depression. As discussed in detail in Chapter 16, both CBD and THC have shown to be effective treatments for symptoms of depression. If you suffer with depression, you can begin with a CBD-dominant product that contains low levels of THC in a sativa strain. If you have reached a dose of 100mg per day and feel CBD is not strong enough to relieve your symptoms, you may need to begin to increase the amount of THC to a 3:1 or 2:1 CBD:THC ratio (20–40mgCBD with 2.5–20mgTHC) until you feel happy and comfortable. We will discuss the systemic benefits of CBD during chemotherapy momentarily, but don't be surprised if you really like the effects of a sativa-based THC vape or edible with little to no CBD. Sativa-based THC products can deliver a much-needed mood boost and mental reprieve from the trials of chemotherapy while at the same time helping to settle a nauseated belly and easing pain, with or without additional CBD.

As always, it is important to determine your optimal dosage of THC when using edibles for either depression or fatigue (see Chapter 3) because too little THC will have no effect at all, and too much THC can cause excessive drowsiness, even when using a sativa product. Inhaled sativa products work quickly and on-demand, which is often preferable for patients. When dealing with fatigue or depression along with anxiety, patients may opt for a slightly more relaxing strain, such as a sativa-dominant hybrid or CBD-dominant sativa strain. These strains can boost the mood while preventing an increase in anxiety which can occur when using a strong THC rich sativa strain.

Nausea and Vomiting (Emesis)

Chemotherapy Induced Nausea and Vomiting (CINV) is an unrelenting condition that can cause patients to lose weight rapidly, putting further treatment at risk. Oral dosing of cannabis can be used to prevent heavy bouts of nausea while inhaled products work best for on-demand relief (highly preferable for many patients) during active emesis.

THC is the cannabinoid shown to be most effective when treating chemotherapy-induced nausea and vomiting.[3] The dorsal vagal complex (DVC) in the brainstem regulates emesis and contains, like the gastrointestinal tract, endocannabinoid receptors upon which cannabinoids exhibit their anti-nausea effects.

An inhaled sativa strain may be adequate to combat nausea, but for more severe episodes of CINV a relaxing hybrid or full indica strain will offer much stronger relief. Indica strains are very relaxing and seem to be most effective at reducing severe nausea and vomiting.

CBD has been shown to have limited value for treating active emesis but may be useful to treat anxiety which can exacerbate nausea.[4]

In my experience, CBD products that do not contain adequate levels of THC are unsuccessful when treating CINV and can actually decrease the appetite further. However, CBD can be useful for patients who cannot tolerate the euphoric effects of THC by creating a more mild-feeling product. When treating severe nausea and vomiting with a combination of THC and CBD, look for strains that have close to equal amounts of each cannabinoid (1:1 CBD:THC). If tolerated, try increasing the levels of THC (1:2 CBD:THC ratio) to increase relief even further. THC-based indica products with little to no CBD are best at stimulating the appetite while calming CINV episodes.

Pain

Pain from cancer can be caused by inflammation, nerve damage, or as a direct result of the cancer growth. For this reason, as discussed in Chapter 8, a combination of THC and CBD is often most successful when treating cancer-related pain.

Severe Pain: THC is extremely effective for pain, especially when used in combination with CBD. Sativex®, a cannabis-derived oral mucosal spray containing equal proportions of THC and CBD, was approved in Canada in 2007 for intractable cancer pain and in the United Kingdom for spasticity due to multiple sclerosis.[5] Patients with severe pain requiring oxycodone or other strong opioids will likely need at least a small amount of THC in their chosen product for adequate pain relief.

Patients should begin with a product that contains a ratio of 3:1 or 2:1 CBD:THC. Edibles may offer better pain relief than inhaled products for chronic pain and should be dosed around the clock every 6–8 hours to prevent pain. It is harder to overcome pain than it is to prevent it, so be sure to treat your pain as needed. Follow the dosing guidelines available in Chapter 3 to dial in your dose. Patients should begin with 2–5mg THC (combined with double or triple the amount of CBD) and increase the dosage by 2.5mg per dose every 24–48 hours until pain is managed.

Moderate Pain: Patients with mild to moderate pain can begin using isolated CBD with little to no THC. A study in the *Journal of British Medicine* found that CBD can actually prevent nerve damage induced by paclitaxel (Taxol), a chemotherapy drug used to treat breast, ovarian, and lung cancer, thus reducing overall pain.[6] I have witnessed countless patients achieve substantial relief from neuropathic pain using just a CBD solution. If CBD does not deliver complete pain relief, a 5:1 or 4:1 CBD:THC can offer more pain relief with little intoxication.

Ideally, when treating pain, you should use something that is non-sedating during the day and something relaxing in the evening. Experiment to find your favorite ratio of CBD to THC in sativa and indica products, both inhaled and as edibles. Again, it is always harder to overcome pain than it is to prevent it (the same is true for nausea), so smaller doses used around the clock are more effective than larger doses taken infrequently. Around the clock dosing also helps patients to develop a tolerance and reduce the intoxicating effects of THC.

Topical Products for Treating Radiation Burns

Radiation treatment uses high energy particles directed at the area of cancer to destroy cancer cells but can damage surrounding healthy tissue in the process. Patients can be left with nerve damage that may or may not heal properly.

Endocannabinoid receptors, specifically CB1-positive cells, have been found at the site of incision wounds in mice 6–14 hours after injury, indicating these receptors are involved in the inflammatory process of the skin and, therefore, may be effectively treated with topical cannabis products.[7]

Cannabinoids exhibit antibacterial, anti-tumor, and antiviral properties while relieving pain and are ideal for burns on the skin due to radiation.[8, 9] Creams and lotions with THC and CBD should be applied as often as needed to treat pain and itch caused by radiation burns and can help accelerate wound healing.

Wounds that aren't healing properly, thus opening the body to infection, can be treated with undiluted, CO_2-extracted cannabis oil as discussed in Chapter 7. One patient I met that had a gaping wound in his chest as a result of thyroid cancer treatment was on the verge of having a muscle extracted and placed over the wound in order to close the hole (ouch!). Instead, he applied a 1:1 CBD:THC oil every 24 hours, and the wound closed beautifully in under three weeks.

Riva

Riva came to the dispensary because of side effects from her breast cancer treatments. When I asked her if she was dealing with any burns from her radiation treatments, she told me she was in pain and itching all night long on her radiation-treated breast. I recommended a THC+CBD cream and told her to apply it whenever the area bothered her. When I caught up with her a few weeks later, she said her oncologist was shocked by how well she was healing and told her to continue whatever she was doing because it was working.

CBD and THC Use for Killing Cancer Cells (RSO)

There is a lot of excitement within the cannabis industry—as well as the oncology community—because of the potential cancer-killing benefits of cannabis. Another drug in the cancer-fighting arsenal that can work synergistically with chemotherapy and with less toxic effects is a welcome change. We already know cannabinoids display anti-tumor and anti-cancer activity, and it's likely that they will be used for cancer treatment in the future. The most effective current chemotherapy regimens work by combining several drugs together for better cancer eradication at lower doses, and research for breast and prostate cancer indicates that cannabis deserves to be on the list of cancer-killing therapies available to patients.

THC has been shown to kill cancer cells for multiple types of cancer, but oral dosing has finite potential at this time because of the well-known strong psychoactive side effects related to high dose THC.[10, 11] Patients who wish to treat cancer with THC will require hundreds of milligrams per day, which is the limiting factor when using cannabis to treat cancer. If you find 10mg of THC a bit strong, imagine how intense a 100mg dose must feel. Slowly and incrementally increasing the dosage with a 1:1 ratio CBD:THC is ideal, but anyone taking such high dosages of THC, even with CBD, will have to deal with strong side effects.

Patients can avoid the euphoria of such extreme doses with rectal administration, but high dose THC suppositories are not widely available in most dispensaries. Patients consuming high dosages of oral THC need to very slowly increase their dose to an effective, cancer-killing level as observed through blood work or scanned images. It can take weeks to achieve a sufficient dose, and costs can be upwards of $1,000 a month, although some producers within the cannabis industry have programs that help defray the costs of such expensive treatments.

CBD displays anticancer qualities for several tumor types, including breast cancer.[12, 13, 14] A 2013 study published in Anticancer Research showed that lower doses of CBD inhibit cell growth and division, while higher concentrations show indications of cell death. This does not mean that patients can simply take higher and higher doses of CBD to kill more cancer cells. (If only it was that easy.)

Greater cytotoxicity was seen within the study when there was a break in treatment. This indicates that "off" periods of treatment, common with chemotherapy, achieve better results than continuous dosing of CBD. Participants in this study saw the greatest benefit when cells were treated with cannabinoids (CBD + CBG) for two days, followed by three drug-free days, and another two days of treatment with CBD and CBG.[15]

It comes as no surprise that studies support the use of multiple cannabinoids used together, backing what cannabis advocates have been arguing for years: Whole plant medicine is preferable to using the isolated THC and CBD molecules.

How CBD May Help Prevent Chemotherapy-Induced Organ Damage

CBD reduces inflammation and inflammatory cytokines and is an antioxidant and a reactive oxygen species (ROS) scavenger.[15] Therefore, supplementing with CBD before, during, and after chemotherapy may help reduce systemic inflammation and organ damage due to toxic chemotherapeutic agents.

	THC Sativa	THC Hybrid	THC Indica	CBD	THC+CBD
Nausea	GOOD	BETTER	BEST	**GOOD:** Must contain a minimum of 50% THC	**DEPENDS:** Good for anxiety induced nausea. Not good for chemotherapy induced nausea
Fatigue	**BEST:** High doses can lead to anxiety or drowsiness. Do not use past 4:00 p.m. if trouble sleeping	**GOOD:** Use a sativa leaning hybrid	**DO NOT USE**	**DEPENDS:** Use sativa based products only	**DEPENDS:** Some products are more relaxing than others. High dose CBD can cause sedation
Joint Pain	GOOD	GOOD	GOOD	**BEST:** For severe joint pain	**BETTER:** Start using alone and add THC if needed
Muscle Spasm	GOOD	BETTER	BEST	**GOOD:** Use product with a minimum of 50% THC	**DO NOT USE**
Increase Appetite	GOOD	**BETTER:** Use more relaxing hybrids	BEST	**GOOD:** Use product with a minimum of 50% THC	**DO NOT USE**
Insomnia	**DO NOT USE**	**GOOD:** Use relaxing hybrids only	BEST	**GOOD:** Use indica based products only	**DEPENDS:** Some products are more relaxing than others

CBD was shown to reduce nephrotoxicity (kidney damage) and improve kidney function when used with cisplatin, a highly nephrotoxic chemotherapeutic drug.[16] In the study, patients were given 2.5mg/kg to 10mg/kg of CBD 90 minutes before cisplatin was administered. The greatest benefits were seen at the highest doses.[17]

CBD can help combat the inflammation and damage caused by chemotherapy without the psychoactive side effects of THC and should, therefore, be considered first-line therapy for all chemotherapy patients to help protect the organs and to reduce the spread of cancer cell.

CHAPTER 10

HIV

"It is a curious fact that the only socially accepted and used drugs known to cause tissue damage (alcohol and tobacco) are the ones whose use Western society sanctions."
Lester Grinspoon M.D.[1]
Author of *Marihuana Reconsidered*

Human Immunodeficiency Virus, or HIV, is a virus that infects and destroys CD4 T-cells of the immune system, thereby reducing the body's ability to fight against infections. HIV.gov reports that about 1.1 million people are infected with HIV and about 15% of those people are unaware that they carry the virus.[2]

HIV is a progressive condition, but patients today receive an excellent prognosis due to the development of multiple pharmaceutical regimens that decrease the virus's ability to replicate itself and reduce the progression of the disease. Unfortunately, medications used to treat HIV infections have significant short term and long term side effects that can make patient compliance a struggle.

In this chapter, I summarize the pharmacology for HIV and show how cannabis can counteract some of the negative side effects associated with these drugs to help patients feel better and remain compliant.

Pharmaceutical Treatments for HIV

Medications designed to treat the HIV virus are among the greatest scientific discoveries of the twentieth century because they have added decades to the lives of people infected with the virus. Unfortunately, this benefit is accompanied by severe, complex side effects that can leave patients feeling sick, discouraged and depressed.

Complex drug regimens for HIV are called **antiretroviral therapy (ART)**. Typical HIV regimens will include three HIV medicines from at least two different drug classes summarized below:

Nucleoside reverse transcriptase inhibitors (NRTIs) block an enzyme that HIV needs to make copies of itself.

Non-nucleoside reverse transcriptase inhibitors (NNRTIs) bind to, and later alter an enzyme that HIV needs to make copies of itself.

Protease inhibitors block another enzyme (protease) that HIV uses to make copies of itself.

Fusion inhibitors block HIV from entering the CD4 T-cells of the immune system (the cells that are destroyed by the virus).

CCR5 antagonists block CCR5 co-receptors on the surface of certain immune cells that HIV needs to enter the cells.

Integrase inhibitors block an enzyme that HIV needs to make copies of itself.

Post attachment inhibitors block CD4 receptors on the surface of the cell where HIV needs to enter.

AIDSinfo.nih.gov lists the common short-term and long term side effects associated with starting an HIV regimen in the chart on page 155.[3]

It's easy to see how compliance with antiretroviral therapy can be a major issue when treating this disease. Patients who experience continual nausea and weakness will find it difficult to remain compliant with the drug therapies. The choice to discontinue antiretroviral therapy inevitably puts their lives at risk. Although medications are highly effective, they will require strict patient adherence in order to work. Just one missed dose of an HIV medication can allow the virus to mutate and become resistant to a patient's current pharmaceutical regimen. Once resistant, patients will need to start all over with a new list of medica-

Short-term side effects include:
- feeling tired
- nausea (upset stomach)
- vomiting
- diarrhea
- headache
- fever
- muscle pain
- occasional dizziness
- insomnia

Long-term side effects include:
- kidney problems, including kidney failure
- liver damage (hepatotoxicity)
- heart disease
- diabetes or insulin resistance
- increased fat levels in the blood (hyperlipidemia)
- changes in how the body uses and stores fat (lipodystrophy)
- weakening of the bones (osteoporosis)
- nerve damage (peripheral neuropathy)
- mental health-related effects, including insomnia, depression, and thoughts of suicide

tions, an exhausting option for many people.

The HIV virus coupled with multiple medications for treatment can induce nausea, weakness, and a decreased appetite leading to a condition called *cachexia*, a loss of muscle and weight that can decrease a patient's ability to maintain good health.

Besides the debilitating physical side effects of the virus and medication therapies, patients live with an emotional stigma from an HIV diagnosis that can lead to depression, anxiety, and a withdrawal from society.

Cannabis Treatments for Symptoms of HIV

Cannabis has been used to help combat symptoms associated with HIV since the virus was first identified back in the 1980s. Mary Jane Rathbun, better known as Brownie Mary, was one of the first cannabis advocates in San Francisco to fight for the right to provide cannabis brownies to patients ravaged by the effects of HIV-AIDS. Patients described how her brownies brought them back from the brink of death.[4]

While cannabis can improve the quality of life for patients living with HIV, a 2008 study showed that the molecule **denbinobin** in cannabis actually inhibits HIV-1 reactivation and may help decrease viral load.[5] This is an exciting discovery that may open the door for the development of future therapeutic targets when treating the virus.

Antiretroviral therapy saves lives, but as we discussed, is difficult to tolerate. A recent study in the *Journal of Acquired Immune Deficiency Syndrome* showed that patients who used cannabis were 3.3 times more likely to adhere to antiviral regimens than patients who did not use cannabis.[6]

Cannabis with THC can be inhaled 30–60 minutes before taking HIV medications to suppress nausea and increase appetite, thus keeping patients compliant with ART and slowing the progression of cachexia. In fact, anytime a patient develops nausea, they can quickly resolve the issue with a puff or two. This kind of relief allows patients to be more productive at work and in life while continuing to adhere to their strict medication regimen.

Cannabis can be used to combat emotional issues associated with an HIV diagnosis, and regimens can be tailored to meet each patient's needs using a combination of cannabinoids and beneficial terpene profiles. As discussed in Chapter 16, CBD and THC can reduce symptoms of anxiety and depression (sativa) and help with stress-induced sleep issues (indica).

Nerve damage from ART can be treated, and possibly prevented, with CBD. The endocannabinoid system is active throughout the central and peripheral nervous systems for reduction of pain and to alleviate neurodegenerative and inflammatory damage.[7, 8] Multiple studies demonstrate CBD's ability to decrease inflammation and neuropathic pain.[9, 10] If you read the previous chapter about using cannabis to combat the side effects of chemotherapy, you know that CBD can help reduce the harmful effects from chemotherapeutic agents that cause organ damage. So, why not apply this knowledge to possibly reduce nerve damage caused by HIV medications? Patients who experience nerve damage or want to prevent it can start a CBD regimen of 20-40mg taken every 6–8 hours. If this dosage is not sufficient for nerve pain relief, patients can follow the guidelines in Chapter 3 for dialing in an effective higher dose.

Neurological complications due to central nervous system damage can lead to headaches, memory loss, issues with balance and coordination, and seizures, all of which may be helped when treated with cannabis. Cannabis strains rich in CBD and low in THC have been used to reduce seizure activity and systemic inflammation, and may offer significant benefits for the many neurological issues associated with HIV disease and treatment. Begin treatment with products that contain a 10:1 to 5:1 CBD:THC ratio (20mg CBD with 2mg THC), then increase THC levels until you're happy with the effects. Sativa strains will feel more clear, wakeful and help with focus during the daytime, while indica strains can help with sleep disorders.

Long-term use of HIV medications can lead to the development of diabetes in some patients. A recent study published in *The American Journal of Medicine* looked at data from a National Health and Nutrition Examination Survey (NHANES) from 2005 and 2010 and found a significant link between the regular use of marijuana and better blood sugar control.[11] (I discuss cannabis and diabetes in Chapter 19.) Cannabis applications for diabetes have yet to be researched, but we do know it works as a powerful anti-inflammatory, and diabetes is the result of the destruction of beta cells in the pancreas due to excess inflammation.

Overall, cannabis offers an interlude from the chronic physical and emotional symptoms from HIV disease and the rigid pharmaceutical treatments. We cannot minimize the emotional toll an HIV diagnosis can take on a person or the comfort cannabis can offer. Peter McWilliams, author, HIV patient, and cannabis advocate wrote, "In addition to its remarkable anti-nausea effects, medical marijuana had one additional benefit–now how do I say this without corrupting the youth of the nation?–I had forgotten how enjoyable it is being stoned. I had forgotten, too, how healing enjoyment can be. Yes, pleasure is therapy. Ease to unravel disease. A deep appreciation of life as an answer to death."[12]

CHAPTER 11

Cannabis for Migraines

*"Not only are there thousands of migraine patients who benefit
from cannabis, but cannabis has been cited by such historical
medical luminaries as Sir William Osler, M.D. (considered the father
of modern medicine) and Dr. Morris Fishbein (long-time editor
of JAMA) as the best treatment for migraines (back in the
days before the Congress ignored the AMA and over the
AMA's objection, passed the Marijuana Tax Act)."*
Dr. David L. Bearman[1]

About 1 out of every 7 Americans will suffer from migraines so severe that words cannot describe the pain.[2] Headache sufferer Emily Dickinson wrote:[3]

Pain has an element of blank
It cannot recollect
When it began—or if there were
A day when it was not.

Current migraine research supports a consensus that migraine pain is caused by a lowering of the threshold of nerve signal processing in response to a release of pro-inflammatory agents, but why this happens remains a mystery.[4] Cannabis is known to affect nerve signaling and has been shown to be effective for both migraine relief and prevention.

Factors contributing to migraines are internal and external, hormonal and environmental. "Cannabinoids—due to their anti-convulsive, analgesic (pain), anti-nausea, and anti-inflammatory effects—present a promising class of compounds for both acute and prophylactic treatment of migraine pain."[5]

In this chapter, I summarize the plethora of pharmaceuticals used to treat migraines and the dangers associated with them. I'll talk about how to use cannabis to treat an emerging migraine, as well as how to help prevent future attacks.

Pharmaceutical Treatments for Migraines

One of the biggest problems migraine sufferers face today is the severe, life-threatening side effects associated with the pharmaceutical solutions available to them, as well as limitations regarding how much a patient can safely take. Pharmacology is limited by maximum allowable doses per day, per week, and per month or risks escalate quickly. These dosage ceilings can leave patients that experience frequent migraines unmedicated during a painful episode.

Current migraine medications include non-steroidal anti-inflammatory drugs (NSAIDs) such as ibuprofen and naproxen, ergotamines, anti-seizure medications, and a class of drugs called triptans. A new class of migraine medications called **CGRP inhibitors** was approved by the FDA in 2019 for chronic migraine sufferers. These drugs already have doctors and pharmacists wondering about their risky, long-term cardiac and pulmonary side effects, along with their whopping price tag estimated to be between $8,500 and $20,000 per year. The true risks associated with CGRPs will not be seen for at least ten years under real life patient conditions. (Migraine sufferers, you're the guinea pigs in this experiment.) CGRP inhibitors are estimated to create a new drug market with up to 10 billion dollars in annual revenues, so drug companies have a strong incentive to expand this lucrative market.

Ergotamines, which work on the sympathetic nervous system in the brain to affect blood flow, were developed at the beginning of the twentieth century and are derived from a fungus.[6] They have been shown to be effective when treating migraines but, as with so many medicines, have significant drug interactions. The number of doses per day and per week are limited, and these medications cannot be taken orally due to break-down in the stomach. They are prescribed today as a nasal spray and are also available by injection.

A class of drugs called **triptans,** beginning with Imitrex (sumatrip-tan) in 1993, changed the game regarding how migraines are treated. Triptans work within the serotonin receptor system, specifically the 5-HT1 serotonin receptor, to shrink swollen blood vessels in the brain, the result of which is migraine resolution. Triptans have become first-line therapy for the treatment of migraines, although they too contain a long list of side effects ranging from mild drowsiness to death. Triptans should not be used by those who have a history of risk factors for heart disease, high blood pressure, high cholesterol, angina, peripheral vas-cular disease, impaired liver function, stroke, or diabetes. This excludes many migraine sufferers. Patients are also limited to the number of mil-ligrams they can take per day, per week, and per month. If they exceed these amounts, they run the risk of developing a life-threatening condi-tion called serotonin syndrome.

Cannabis Treatments for Migraines and the Prevention of Migraines

The use of cannabis for migraine prevention and resolution has been documented since 1840.[7] Cannabis provides anti-inflammatory action through the endocannabinoid system using CB2 receptors found in the periphery and CB1 receptors of the central nervous system. A re-cently established hypothesis, the Clinical Endocannabinoid Deficiency (CECD) hypothesis, looks at the endocannabinoid system's role in mi-graine prevention and its contribution to overall mental and physical health and wellbeing.[8, 9] It is thought that a deficiency in cannabinoids, anandamide and 2-AG, creates an imbalance in the body that leads to the development of chronic disease, including migraines. Cannabis can be used as a supplement to maintain homeostasis, decrease inflammation, and offer a resolution of symptoms with low toxicity.

A 2016 study of Colorado patients who suffered with chronic migraines found that those who began using cannabis, either preventatively or to treat an active migraine, were able to reduce the number of migraines they had per month by more than 50% with positive effects being reported in almost 40% of participants.[10] These are impressive numbers for any medicine, much less one that has been around for thousands of years.

Prevention of chronic migraines can be accomplished by medicating with cannabis at regular intervals throughout the day. Strains or products rich in CBD combined with lower levels of THC are best, although many patients can still achieve measurable relief with CBD-isolated products or THC dominant strains. Micro-dosing, as discussed in Chapter 3, is an effective tool for reducing the number of monthly migraines in chronic migraine sufferers. Patients should slowly and systematically increase their oral dosage of THC (start with 1mg every 8 to 12 hours), combined with higher doses of CBD (10-20mg every 8 to 12 hours), until maximum effectiveness is reached with minimal intoxication. As always, more cannabinoids are not necessarily more effective, so aim for that sweet spot in dosing. Lower doses of multiple cannabinoids may be more effective than higher doses of a single cannabinoid.

Patients who prefer to inhale should medicate at regular intervals throughout the day (every 6–8 hours) to keep cannabinoid levels in the blood consistent. Journaling can help patients determine the optimal timing of dosages, but a minimum of two doses a day is likely to be required.

Acute episodes of migraines are treated differently than preventative therapy. Once a migraine begins, it is important to stop the cascade of inflammatory events that lead to a severe, crippling migraine. At the first sign of a migraine, patients should take a moderate to large oral dose of CBD (25–50mg) with or without additional THC (as tolerated) since THC helps to relax tight muscles and further reduce inflammation to help resolve the migraine. Patients may not be able to medicate with

THC if a migraine comes on at work or while driving. Follow the initial loading dose of CBD with a second dose (25–50mg) 4 to 6 hours later and every 4–6 hours until resolved.

While waiting for the oral dose of CBD to begin working, patients can begin to resolve painful symptoms by inhaling strains rich in CBD with moderate to high levels of THC (2:1 or 1:1 CBD:THC). Be aware of your overall THC intake (oral and inhaled) to avoid excessive consumption. It's important for patients to realize, higher doses of cannabis are required during an active migraine. Patients who have not had oral CBD available at the onset of a migraine report that they are still able to find relief by inhaling relatively large amounts of a 2:1 or 1:1 CBD:THC ratio every 10–15 minutes. Once you feel the migraine starts to resolve, you can begin to back off on your treatment.

Mary

One Tuesday morning, our dispensary receptionist was wearing sunglasses and a hoodie with the hood pulled up. She looked like she wanted to curl up and die. When I asked her what happened, she said she had been suffering from a migraine for the last three days and could not afford to take any more days off. I gave her a 25mg dose of CBD from a dropper of pure oil I always keep on hand in my bag. (As a pharmacist, I'm always prepared with a medication for something.) She swallowed the dose and we went on with the busy day.

After 3 or 4 hours, I went to check on her and found her sitting up, no longer wearing her sunglasses. I asked how she felt, and she said that she was feeling a bit better. I gave her another 25mg dose of CBD oil. By the end of the workday, she said the migraine was gone.

Cannabis has historically been extremely successful at preventing and treating migraines and, when legalized on a federal level, will take its rightful place as a safe, first-line treatment for migraine prevention and cure.

When treating a migraine, look for strains and products that are rich in CBD because of the strong anti-inflammatory effects. Remember, too, that THC can play an important role in resolution of acute migraines by decreasing pain and promoting relaxation. Whatever products you choose, medicate regularly, and don't be afraid to increase your dosage during an active migraine until you observe maximum benefit.

CHAPTER 12

Multiple Sclerosis (MS)

"Cannabinoids are now known to have the capacity for neuromodulation, via direct, receptor-based mechanisms, at numerous levels within the nervous system. These provide therapeutic properties that may be applicable to the treatment of neurological disorders, including anti-oxidative, neuroprotective effects, analgesia, anti-inflammatory actions, immunomodulation, modulation of glial cells and tumor growth regulation. Beyond that, the cannabinoids have also been shown to be remarkably safe with no potential for overdose."

Gregory T. Carter, MD[1]

Clinical Professor at the School of Medicine at the University of Washington and co-director of the Muscular Dystrophy Association (ALS) Center

Multiple sclerosis symptoms are mostly felt and often not seen. An MS sufferer might look good on the outside, while his body is throwing a fit on the inside.

Multiple sclerosis (MS) was first recognized in 1868 by French neurologist Jean-Martin Charcot who was able to link a peculiar set of symptoms to plaques found in the brain.[2] MS is a dysfunction of the human immune response in which our own T-cells attack the myelin coating that runs along the nerve cells of the central nervous system, resulting in what's known as demyelination. As the myelin breaks down, nerve signals cannot conduct smoothly along the full length of the nerve, so patients develop symptoms such as brain fog, muscle spasms, muscle weakness, numbness, optic nerve damage, bowel issues and difficulty with walking and muscle coordination. MS is a progressive disease, and its cause remains unknown.

More than 2.3 million people are diagnosed with MS worldwide, but diagnostic challenges and a lack of a national registry make it difficult to have an accurate number of MS patients.[3] The progression of the disease is unpredictable, and some forms of MS are more aggressive than others. A lack of muscle control due to decreased nerve conduction leads to difficulty driving and the inability to work, which inevitably leads to additional financial and emotional strain. MS is typically diagnosed in patients between the ages of 20 and 40. The progression of the disease is unique to each patient. Prognosis may be influenced by diet, stress, pharmaceutical medications, alternative therapies, and genetics. I have met with dozens of MS patients; no two patients have the exact same symptoms. In this chapter we will discuss the pharmacology for treating MS and how cannabis can be used for symptom relief and to possibly affect underlying disease progression.

Jane and Bill

Working in a cannabis dispensary, you are bound to have at least one patient almost every day who is suffering from MS. I will never forget the day I had two patients, each with MS diagnoses made over 20 years prior, who had two completely different experiences.

The first patient was a woman in her late forties. Jane arrived in a wheelchair, was losing her eyesight, and was suffering from debilitating pain and muscle spasms every day. She was on a regimen of Copaxone, gabapentin, baclofen, and opioids for her pain but could barely use her hands and was severely depressed due to her current state of health. The baclofen was barely effective for her muscle spasms and the opioids left her feeling exhausted and exacerbated the constipation brought on by the MS itself. Jane was unfamiliar with cannabis but, over time, was able to decrease all her medications and felt less pain and experienced fewer spasms overall.

The second patient I saw later that day was a gentleman in his fifties that, from all appearances, looked perfectly healthy. He had chosen a more homeopathic route after his diagnosis. He'd been a regular cannabis user since college and had begun bee venom therapy almost immediately after his MS diagnosis. I knew bees did amazing things for our planet but had not yet heard of them being used as a treatment for multiple sclerosis. He described how he would administer bee stings along a meridian (a nerve center) in a way that's similar to what is used in acupuncture twice a week. He ordered his bees through the mail. (Can you imagine?) He had begun with one bee sting twenty years ago and was, at the time we talked, up to 10–12 stings per treatment. He had seen a very little progression of the disease and was on no prescription medications. I was absolutely fascinated at the differences in the progression of the disease between these two patients.

Pharmaceutical Treatments for Multiple Sclerosis

There is a myriad of symptoms that accompany an MS diagnosis, but the most common type of MS, and the one that most MS specific prescription medications are designed for, is relapsing-remitting MS (RRMS). Patients with a RRMS diagnosis experience disease remission (a lessening of symptoms) followed by symptom "flares" that can last for weeks to months. Flares, also known as attacks or relapses, increase myelin damage leading to symptom progression and a permanent increase in the severity of symptoms. Flares are treated with high-dose corticosteroids such as prednisone and methylprednisolone. These drugs have powerful side effects, especially when taken for weeks or months at a time, a common occurrence during a flare.

Pharmacology focuses on decreasing the frequency of flares and slowing disease progression. The most commonly prescribed drugs are classified as **Disease-Modifying Therapy (DMT)**. The goal of prescribing these drugs is to reduce the frequency and severity of relapses over time. Studies show that they are most effective when started immediately after diagnosis.

A 2016 report from Pennsylvania State University compared delayed therapy to continuing therapy of Copaxone, one of the first DMT drugs to come to market in 1997.[4] The report found Copaxone caused a shift from auto-aggressive pro-inflammatory Th1 cells to protective anti-inflammatory Th2 cells, which migrated into the central nervous system providing improved long-term benefits and significant decrease in disease progression.[5] Patients may not see a benefit immediately, but studies such as these show DMT provides overall long-term benefits.

The biggest issue is that DMT is expensive. Very expensive. According to an analysis published in 2017 by the Institute for Clinical and Economic Review (ICER), the annual cost of medications for MS range from $63,000 to nearly $104,000, so the financial burden of an MS diagnosis is substantial.[6] A study on the pricing of DMT therapies found first generation DMT therapy that originally cost $8,000–$11,000 now cost over $60,000. Same medication, higher price every year. DMT medication prices have increased at a higher rate than any other class of medications on the market.[7]

Along with disease-modifying drugs, patients with MS are given a long list of other medications to combat symptoms. Baclofen and other muscle relaxants are standard therapies for muscle spasms, along with neuropathic agents such as gabapentin and pregabalin (Lyrica). Opioids and non-steroidal anti-inflammatories (NSAIDs) are prescribed for additional pain, which, when mixed, can leave patients struggling with fatigue and over sedation.

Along with the cocktail of meds to treat the symptoms of MS, side effects from DMT therapies can be difficult to manage. Anxiety, joint pain, muscle stiffness, and depression are common. Because the benefits of continuing therapies seem to outweigh the risks, patients are left overwhelmed by both the diagnosis and the treatments. It is at this time, when they are drowning in pills, that patients will turn to alternative treatments such as cannabis to help decrease side effects from their current drug profile and alleviate symptoms of the underlying disease.

Cannabis Treatments for Multiple Sclerosis

Cannabis is a medicine that's known to treat multiple symptoms simultaneously. It can decrease muscle spasms while increasing muscle tone and bladder control, and can even help patients achieve a better sex life (bonus!).

With all we know about cannabis and the endocannabinoid system, is it possible that cannabis is helping with just the symptoms of MS, or can it actually be helping to slow the progression of the underlying disease by aligning an aspect of the endocannabinoid system that was once off-balance?

In 1994, researchers conducted an experiment in which guinea pigs were injected with experimental autoimmune encephalitis (EAE), which is used as a model for MS in a laboratory setting. *All* animals exposed to the disease and treated with a placebo developed the disease, and 98% died as a result. When animals were treated with Δ-9-THC, 95% survived and developed little to no symptoms, and on inspection their brain tissue was less inflamed.[8] As mentioned in the chapter on migraines, the Clinical Endocannabinoid Deficiency (CECD) hypothesis proposes that a lack of cannabinoids can lead to chronic and exacerbated disease, MS being one of them.[9] This approach could substantially change the way MS is treated from the day of diagnosis.

Cannabis for Combating MS Symptoms and Pharmaceutical Side Effects

Powerful corticosteroids are prescribed whenever we need to substantially decrease the body's inflammatory response. From poison ivy to asthma to cancer, steroids have potent anti-inflammatory actions coupled with strong side effects. When used for under two weeks, steroids can cause weight gain, edema, agitation, and sleep disturbances, but are generally safe for most people. When steroids are prescribed during an MS flare, patients can remain on the drug for weeks to months at a time, and side effects can egregiously interfere with normal body functions.

Long-term use of steroids can lead to the development of diabetes, upset stomach and ulceration, glaucoma, nausea and vomiting, headache, insomnia, depression, and anxiety. If we could find another way to decrease chronic inflammation while preventing these nasty side effects, we would really be on to something.

If we look at CBD as a possible alternative, it possesses potent anti-inflammatory properties that may someday allow patients to decrease dosages of steroid treatments. I have witnessed several MS patients who could not tolerate another dose of a steroid and instead used high-dose CBD (100mg) in place of prescription steroid treatments with equivalent results. The biggest downside of this therapy is the cost. CBD therapy currently costs much, much more than the average prescription for a corticosteroid.

Muscle spasms due to damaged and inflamed nerves can be severe in MS patients. Baclofen, a centrally acting muscle relaxant, is the most commonly prescribed medication to treat these painful muscle spasms. As is the case with many older pharmaceuticals, how baclofen works is not exactly understood, but the benefits are limited by dosage. Too high a dose and patients can experience muscle weakness and extreme dizziness, while too low a dose offers minimal spasm relief. By adding cannabis (THC and CBD) to an MS drug regimen, patients can often decrease baclofen dosages to more comfortable levels while still experiencing powerful relief.

Sativex is a plant-based 1:1 CBD:THC oral spray that is sold as an adjunct therapy for MS spasticity in Canada, the United Kingdom, Australia, and Spain. Each dose delivers about 2.5mg of THC and CBD. A double blind, placebo-controlled study found that "Sativex was significantly superior to placebo for spasm frequency and sleep disruption."[10] It is a shame MS patients in the United States are unable to use this medication like the rest of the world due to federal scheduling of THC.

Strains of cannabis used to treat muscle spasms should include THC, an antispasmodic, but the freedom to choose the amount of THC lies with the patient. I find indica-dominant hybrids or full indica strains to be most effective for muscle relaxation, but they do cause substantially more drowsiness and sedation than sativa-dominant strains. Patients can begin using a hybrid strain first, during the daytime, then move to a more sedating product if they need to relax their muscles more.

Patients who need to treat severe muscle spasms should look for products that combine CBD and THC in a 1:1, 2:1, or 3:1 CBD:THC ratio. Products can be chosen based on the immediate need to alleviate symptoms. Use more THC when spasms and pain increase and lower amounts of THC when symptoms subside.

For quick, on-demand relief, patients can use inhalation or sublingual dosing. Oral formulations should be dosed every 6–12 hours around the clock if being used for prevention, although some patients use edibles every 4 hours during a flare. High, frequent dosing of THC can lead to excessive drowsiness. Products for MS patients will ideally be low in sugar and gluten-free because some studies suggest both compounds exacerbate inflammation.

Nerve pain is most often treated with gabapentin, pregabalin (Lyrica) or duloxetine (Cymbalta). Because CBD is a potent anti-inflammatory and has been shown to be effective when treating nerve pain, it can be used synergistically to treat pain and reduce dosages of gabapentin and pregabalin (Lyrica), or as a total replacement for these medications if they are not well tolerated by patients.[11] CBD has the added benefit of reducing THC euphoria to make it more tolerable for daytime use.

Fatigue is a common complaint heard from MS patients, and the uplifting qualities of a wakeful sativa strain can help with both fatigue and depression. If a full sativa strain causes any anxiety, consider a sativa-dominant hybrid strain such as Jack Herrer or Blue Dream. These strains are wakeful but a bit more relaxing, so they are good for patients that deal with anxiety. Sativa strains such as MediHaze or Harlequin are rich in CBD and great for reducing pain and daytime fatigue while also reducing anxiety.

Injection site swelling from DMT medications can be treated with CBD+THC topical lotions. Use the strongest formulation you can find, and apply it as often as needed until the inflammation subsides.

For additional information on the best strains for your specific symptoms, refer to the chart on page 173 or use the Leafly app.

	THC Sativa	THC Hybrid	THC Indica	CBD
Fatigue	**BEST**	**GOOD:** Use sativa leaning hybrid	**DO NOT USE**	**DEPENDS:** Some products are more relaxing than others. High dose CBD can cause sedation.
Muscle Spasms	**GOOD**	**BETTER:** Use indica leaning hybrid	**BEST**	**DEPENDS:** Use product with minimum of 50% THC
Nerve Pain	**BETTER:** Use product with minimum 50% CBD	**GOOD:** Use product with minimum 50% CBD	**GOOD:** Use product with minimum 50% CBD	**BEST:** Use alone or combine with THC for severe pain
Muscle Weakness	**BETTER**	**BEST:** Use less sedating hybrids	**GOOD:** Use less sedating indica products	**DEPENDS:** Use alone or combine with 50% THC
Sexual Dysfunction	**BETTER**	**BEST:** Use less sedating hybrids	**GOOD:** Use less sedating indica products	**NO EFFECT**
Depression	**BEST:** Use alone or combine with CBD	**GOOD:** Use sativa leaning hybrid	**DO NOT USE**	**GOOD:** Use alone or combine with sativa THC
Cognitive Issues	**BEST:** Use low dose alone or combine with CBD	**GOOD:** Use sativa leaning hybrid	**DEPENDS:** Drowsiness can lead to confusion	**BEST:** Use alone or combine with sativa THC

Ganja:
a Hindi word for
the hemp plant.

CHAPTER 13

Alzheimer's Disease (AD)

*"THC and its analogues may provide an improved therapeutic for
Alzheimer's disease [by] simultaneously treating both
the symptoms and progression of Alzheimer's disease."*
Lisa M. Eubanks, PhD[1]
Staff Scientist at the Scripps Research Institute and
the Skaggs Institute for Chemical Biology

Alzheimer's disease (AD), along with other forms of dementia, affects one in three seniors, and the number of patients diagnosed has increased 145% between 2000 and 2017. In 1906, Dr. Alois Alzheimer noted changes in the brain tissue of a woman who had memory loss, trouble speaking, and exhibited unpredictable behavior. Upon analysis, her brain showed bundled nerve fibers and plaques (now called amyloid plaques) that, along with a loss of connection between neurons, are still among the main indicators used to establish an Alzheimer's diagnosis today.[2]

There are several types of dementia diagnoses that correspond to the location of the sticky, protein beta-amyloid plaques in the brain and are also based on patient symptoms. Damage to the brain can start up to ten years before symptoms even begin to appear, so prevention of plaque formation is essential to slow disease progression.[3]

AD begins with mild cognitive impairment, such as forgetting easily remembered information or having difficulty judging how long it will take to complete a task, like driving to a friend's house. Personality changes begin to appear where patients become more withdrawn and tend to easily lose motivation to complete tasks. As damage continues to advance, patients develop drastic personality changes (increased fear and aggression), may lose the ability to communicate, and their muscles become stiff and rigid making it hard to sit or walk. Emotional fluctuations along with physical limitations can place an enormous amount of stress on family and caregivers.

Neurologists and researchers have not identified an underlying cause of Alzheimer's disease, but most believe that systemic, chronic inflammation plays a pivotal role in contributing to tissue damage and impairment of neurologic functions.[4, 5] As discussed in the chapter on pain, currently, we do not have a single, safe pharmaceutical medication designed to treat chronic, systemic inflammation.

AD pharmacology is designed to improve memory or slow disease progression, but current therapies produce limited benefits and carry substantial toxic side effects. On the flip side, cannabis is non-toxic, has an excellent safety profile, and demonstrates neuroprotective and anti-inflammatory effects.[6] With further research, cannabis may just be an important piece of the puzzle to stop the advancement of this brutal disease. Pharmaceutical and cannabis therapies are discussed and compared throughout this chapter.

Pharmaceutical Treatments for Alzheimer's Disease

Pharmacotherapy for preventing and treating AD is extremely limited, which is frustrating for patients and caregivers considering its prevalence in older adults. Current treatments target two areas of the brain:

• **Acetylcholinesterase inhibitors** prevent an enzyme in the brain from breaking down acetylcholine, resulting in higher enzyme levels and better communication between nerve cells.

• **NMDA receptor antagonists** block the activity of the N-methyl-D-aspartate receptor (NMDAR) to decrease levels of glutamate in order to prevent cell death in brain tissues. Glutamate is the major excitatory neurotransmitter in the brain, and excess levels have been linked to chronic neurodegenerative disease.[7]

Four acetylcholinesterase inhibitors are approved in the United States to improve memory in patients with mild to moderate Alzheimer's disease: galantamine, donepezil, tacrine, and rivastigmine, although tacrine is rarely used due to toxic effects in the liver. These drugs can slightly delay the loss of brain function in early disease, but have activity-limiting side effects, including nausea, vomiting, and dizziness.

A study comparing the effectiveness of all four acetylcholinesterase inhibitors when combined with the use of memantine (Namenda), a widely prescribed NMDA receptor antagonist, showed that the greatest benefit at twenty-four weeks was actually observed when patients used an over the counter supplement called Huperazine A. Huperazine A has acetylcholinesterase inhibiting effects and is derived from a plant called the Chinese club moss. It has shown a promising safety profile in phase II trial patients with mild to moderate Alzheimer's disease, and no patients had to withdraw from the study due to adverse effects when Huperazine A was combined with Namenda.[8]

Overstimulation of the NMDA membrane receptors has been implicated as one of the key factors contributing to neuronal injury and cell death. **NMDA receptor antagonists** can either partially or fully block the NMDA receptor. Their efficacy is questionable because NMDA receptor activity is required for normal functioning of the human body, and only drugs that partially block the receptor are clinically acceptable, with memantine (Namenda) being a drug that partially blocks the receptor.

NMDA receptor antagonists are not exclusively used to reduce neurological degeneration in dementia-type diseases. The most common NMDA antagonists are found as an over the counter cough suppressant, dextromethorphan (DXM), as well as the anesthetic and antidepressant ketamine, and the street drug, phencyclidine (PCP). These drugs induce a state of *dissociative anesthesia* that can produce hallucinations, confusion, and behavior changes. These are also listed as possible side effects from NMDA receptor antagonists used to treat Alzheimer's disease.

The most widely prescribed NMDA receptor antagonist has been Namenda, which reached sales of $1.5 billion in 2013–2014 and went off patent in 2015.[9] Memantine (Namenda) was originally used to treat Parkinson's disease, but further research showed that it is an noncompetitive open-channel blocker that has a shorter dwell time on receptors. Shortening the dwell time limits the activity of the NMDA receptor while sparing normal synaptic activity.[10,11,12] These mechanisms help make it an effective treatment for AD with an acceptable side effect profile.

Both classes of drugs used to treat Alzheimer's disease, acetylcholinesterase inhibitors and NMDA receptor antagonists, offer limited benefits for treating symptoms in patients with moderate to advanced AD. As damage progresses and brain functions diminish, patients can exhibit personality changes such as aggression and fearfulness. Pharmaceuticals such as antidepressants, anxiolytics, and anti-psychotics designed to treat behavioral changes in healthy patients are often unsuccessful in patients with Alzheimer's disease and have been linked to increased mortality in patients with dementia.[13]

When we compare these limitations to cannabis, cannabinoid therapy has shown great promise for neuronal protection, while decreasing neuronal damage, and can be used to treat emotional symptoms as well. Cannabis, with its strong anti-inflammatory effects, offers a new therapeutic approach to treating Alzheimer's disease with a preferable side effect profile. A big advantage to using cannabis over pharmaceuticals is the ability to administer it during the most severe stages of disease when pharmacology treatment is limited.

Cannabis Treatments for Alzheimer's Disease

Alzheimer's disease is widespread, progressive, and no currently available pharmaceutical treatments slow the progression of the disease. If you have read the previous chapters on pain and migraines, you know by now that CBD has both potent antioxidant and anti-inflammatory effects on the brain, things that can slow progression of disease.[14] THC is also neuroprotective and can increase levels of acetylcholinesterase that affect amyloid (plaque) production, a key indicator of Alzheimer's disease progression.[15, 16]

The bottom line? A propaganda that touts cannabis as being harmful to the brain is flat out false. In fact, the opposite is true. Cannabis may be the one drug *not* on pharmacy shelves that actually protects and heals the damaged and inflamed Alzheimer's brain while simultaneously assisting with emotional and physical symptoms.

Patients with moderate to severe neurological damage may have trouble remembering to use inhaled or sublingual products (although they may appreciate the fast relief), therefore long-acting oral formulations may be ideal. Oral doses can be scheduled at 8–12-hour intervals to keep patients comfortable around the clock. If a patient becomes more combative and does not want to take a pill, delicious edibles may be an easier way to medicate them. Infused honey can be put into coffee or tea, infused butter or coconut oil can be spread on toast (although it doesn't taste very good), and just about any baked good can be turned into a medicated snack. Caregivers can relax knowing that if they do accidentally give too much or duplicate a dose (common mistakes) their loved one is safe due to the very low toxicity of cannabis.

Ideal products for treating Alzheimer's disease include both THC and CBD, although caregivers may wish to first try CBD alone to see if any benefit is observed. If using CBD alone, I would suggest a starting dose of 20–25mg CBD (10mg if sensitive to medications) every 6 hours. If a 50-100mg dose of CBD around the clock is not producing a significant benefit after two weeks, consider adding THC at a dose of 2–5mg. (See Chapter 3 for dosing CBD and THC.) More aggressive behaviors may need higher doses of indica-based THC.

Products differ between dispensaries, so choosing just one product to start using for AD is overwhelming. A ratio of 10:1 CBD:THC will deliver a 20mg CBD dose with 2–3mg THC and can be a perfect starting point for many AD patients. To keep it simple, begin with any product that contains a lot of CBD and a small amount of THC (10:1 to 5:1 CBD:THC ratio at doses 20mg CBD with 2–4mg THC) and slowly move towards a 2:1 or 1:1 CBD:THC (20–40mg CBD with 10mg THC) product or strain. There is no exact formula, it's what works best for the patient.

Products with a 1:1 or 2:1 CBD:THC ratio may be more helpful at stimulating appetite and decreasing aggression thanks to the higher levels of THC. Caregivers will likely need to experiment with different CBD:THC ratios to find the most effective ratio at reducing negative behaviors without producing excess sedation. If patients are sleeping too much, decrease the THC dose by 25%.

Since THC is a neuroprotectant and anti-inflammatory molecule on its own, there is no reason THC can't be given without CBD, if needed, to stimulate the appetite further or if the CBD seems to be causing a decrease in appetite. The right dose of THC should have patients feeling relaxed, happy, and hungry, but not too sleepy.

Sublingual sprays and film slips work faster than oral products and can be used to calm an anxious or combative patient. A few drops under the tongue or on the inside of the cheek will begin working within 5 to 20 minutes and can last for 3–4 hours.

Sativa products may provide benefits to people who suffer from daytime fatigue and depression thanks to their uplifting qualities and clear-headed feeling. If anxiety develops, switch to a more relaxing strain, such as a sativa-dominant hybrid or full, balanced hybrid. Sativa strains rich in CBD with lower levels of THC can also help with fatigue and depression.

For patients who are agitated or aggressive, consider strains that offer substantial relaxation, such as a hybrid or even a mild indica strain. In my experience, CBN (cannabinol) can be relaxing for many patients and used as a mild anxiolytic. Recreational cannabis products that include

CBN are marketed for sleep, but can also be used to calm an unhappy or aggressive patient.

Cannabis can seem overwhelming on paper, but once you begin to understand how CBD *feels* and THC *feels* it comes into focus quickly. These are safe drugs, so there is little risk of harm when the doses are kept low, as described in this book. I am always available at SwayInnovations.com for questions.

If comfortable, sample some products right away with low levels of THC (1–3mg) to see if it offers any benefit. For very mild symptoms, a good, quality CBD product at an adequate dosage may be all you need. Hemp Gummies are sold online (TribeCBD.com) and offer a respectable 10mg CBD per gummy in a natural, gummy base. Follow your instincts on where to begin. Purchase small quantities of new products to test them before investing in larger quantities. In about two to three weeks you will be able to determine which combinations of CBD and THC are most effective for the most pronounced symptoms. All cannabis is good cannabis for the injured dementia brain, so there is no wrong place to start when medicating with cannabis.

Cotton mouth: the
experience of having
an extremely dry
mouth after consuming
cannabis.

CHAPTER 14

Parkinson's Disease (PD)

"I believe that a federal policy that prohibits physicians
from alleviating suffering by prescribing marijuana for seriously ill
patients is misguided, heavy-handed, and inhumane."
Jerome P. Kassirer, MD[1]
former editor of *The New England Journal of Medicine*

Parkinson's disease (PD) is the second most common neurodegenerative disorder following Alzheimer's disease, although not everyone with Parkinson's disease-like symptoms will receive a diagnosis of Parkinson's disease.[2] Essential tremor, a mild tremor originating in the hands, is a condition that has a much slower progression than Parkinson's disease and is not an indication that patients will eventually develop PD. Katherine Hepburn, for instance, had essential tremors and voice disturbances throughout much of her later life and until her death at age ninety-two without ever experiencing more severe symptoms of PD.

Lab work and brain scans do not aid a Parkinson's diagnosis. PD develops with the destruction of dopamine-producing neurons in an area of the brain called substantia nigra. Damaging protein deposits (Lewy bodies) build up in the brain and are similar to those found in Alzheimer's patients.

Lewy body dementia is the second most common type of progressive dementia and includes Parkinson's-like symptoms such as rigidity and tremors so, in reality, Alzheimer's and Parkinson's disease overlap as conditions of excessive inflammation in the brain that lead to progressive neurological damage. The location of the damage in the brain determines the specific symptoms of either PD or Alzheimer's disease.

Parkinson's disease is a progressive disease of five stages, including motor and non-motor symptoms. Patients in Stage 1 of the disease experience mild symptoms such as a slight tremor on one side of the body with little impaired movement, a decrease in eye blinking, or a lack of swinging arm movements when walking. As the disease progresses, patients may experience painful muscle rigidity, a loss of smell and taste, constipation, or difficulty moving until patients are unable to care for themselves and experience psychosis and hallucinations.

Late-stage Parkinson's disease is brutal for both patient and caregiver. A small amount of hope may be available through the proper use of cannabis. In this chapter, I share pharmacology treatments for PD along with the best way to use cannabis for treating specific PD symptoms.

Pharmaceutical Treatments for Parkinson's Disease

Parkinson's treatment, like all pharmacology for inflammatory neurological conditions, is limited in its effectiveness for easing symptoms and, once again, does not slow disease progression. Pharmaceutical treatment options for PD focus on increasing the amount of dopamine within the brain to reduce symptoms because dopamine-producing cells are the ones that are destroyed over time. The gold standard of treatment for PD is a drug called carbidopa/levodopa (Sinemet), which converts into dopamine once it enters the brain, but can also cause excessive dyskinesias (uncontrolled twisting or excessive movements). As dopamine is depleted in the brain of a person with Parkinson's disease, patients experience depression, a lack of pleasure and motivation, fatigue, sleep disturbances, loss of motor control, and impulsive or destructive behaviors. As damage to the brain continues, the joy of life is expunged, and caring for the patient can become increasingly stressful. Although there is a long list of drugs to treat PD, as you will see, their benefits are offset by dangerous side effects and limited benefit potential.

DOPA decarboxylase inhibitor with dopamine precursor, specifically carbidopa/levodopa (Sinemet), is the most commonly prescribed medication for the treatment of PD symptoms. Levodopa is converted into dopamine once it crosses the blood-brain barrier. Although Sinemet works well for PD symptoms, 30% of patients will suffer side affects that effect motor control within only twenty-four months of initiating therapy.[3] Excessive movements (dyskinesia) are common with this treatment and can draw unwanted attention to a patient's condition. High protein meals can interfere with the absorption of levodopa.

COMT inhibitors block the catechol-O-methyltransferase (COMT) enzyme to prevent the breakdown of levodopa, increasing the amount of dopamine available in the brain. They are useful when treating motor symptoms, but their effectiveness can diminish over time. COMT inhibitors have a long list of side effects that include behavior and mood changes, hallucinations, fatigue, and upset stomach.

Dopamine agonists such as ropinirole (Requip), pramipexole (Mirapex), and rotigotine (Neupro) mimic the dopamine molecule and bind to the dopamine receptor. Dopamine itself cannot be given as an oral pharmaceutical medication because it is destroyed before reaching the brain. Dopamine agonists can be combined with carbidopa/levodopa to help with movement disorders, but the combination can sometimes work against patients. Side effects include nausea, hallucinations, sleep disorders, and dizziness as well as compulsive behaviors such as excessive gambling. If patients develop compulsive behaviors, the medication should be discontinued.

MAO-B inhibitors prevent the breakdown of dopamine by blocking an enzyme called monoamine oxidase. The biggest issue with this class of drugs is not the side effects, although they include dizziness, hallucinations, and upset stomach, but rather the long list of severe drug interactions that include everything from the tyramine in hot dogs and bacon, to cough suppressants.

Anticholinergic drugs (benztropine and trihexyphenidyl) are not

THE CANNABIS PRESCRIPTION

the most effective drugs for treating PD, but they can be used as a secondary treatments for tremors. (They do not, however, help with muscle stiffness.) They are not recommended for older patients because they can cause confusion and memory problems. Unfortunately, they have the common side effects of many drugs: dry mouth, urinary retention, and constipation.

Amantadine was accidentally found to help with PD symptoms.[4] It may mimic dopamine in the brain but was originally used as an antiviral treatment for influenza. It is typically used as an early treatment for PD and can be helpful with dyskinesias.

These drugs will not alter the progression of disease; they are for symptomatic treatments only. Because Parkinson's disease symptoms are both seen (motor) and unseen (emotional), finding an effective treatment poses a challenge. Pharmaceutical medications that are initially successful at reducing motor symptoms can cause substantial dyskinesias due to excess levodopa in the brain. As patients continue to use carbidopa/levodopa, it will, unfortunately, become less and less effective. Some patients find that pills only provide relief for up to two hours at a time.

In the later stages of PD, hallucinations and relentless physical symptoms develop and, in a cruel twist, it is at this time when all PD medications except levodopa (to help with movement) should be discontinued. Note that high doses of levodopa can also lead to hallucinations. Patients with advanced disease may receive anti-psychotics and supportive care for anxiety, depression, and sleep disturbances. Little reprieve is available through pharmaceutical intervention as patients continue to decline.

Cannabis Treatments for Parkinson's Disease

Since the discovery of the Endocannabinoid Receptor System in the early 1990s, research has focused on what effects are mitigated through this massively abundant receptor system. Regulation of motor control is due, in part, to the participation of CB1-related mechanisms in the brain, thus opening the door for cannabinoid therapy that affects motor control in Parkinson's patients.[5] Emotional disturbances, pain, and depression have also been linked to the functions of the endocannabinoid system. This allows cannabis to be used, once again, to treat multiple symptoms simultaneously in order to improve the overall happiness of the patient.

An observational study of almost four hundred patients with PD in Colorado revealed that of the 25% of patients with symptoms who had consumed cannabis almost half proclaimed benefits.[6]

If you want to see for yourself the benefits cannabis can have on a patient with advanced Parkinson's disease, watch the YouTube videos of ex-cop Larry Smith.[7] His erratic movements and voice tremors disappear in under 5 minutes after a few drops of cannabis oil is placed under his tongue. It is astounding to watch.

Cannabis was legalized for medical use in Colorado in 2000 and recreational use in 2014.[8] This created an optimal research environment to discover the benefits of cannabis therapies. Between November 2012 and August 2013, a self-administered study was given to patients at the University of Colorado Hospital Movement Disorders Clinics as well as PD support groups in the Denver metro area to provide information on the effectiveness of complementary and alternative therapy for PD patients.

The survey revealed that many patients used alternative therapies for their movement disorders, but out of the 207 patients who completed the survey only 4.3% reported using cannabis as an alternative treatment. I believe the lack of patient use is due to a lack of patient awareness and education, the exact reason I wrote this book. Other therapies used were vitamins (66%), prayer (59%), massage (45%), and relaxation (32%). While fewer respondents reported using cannabis, it was reported to be the most successful of all alternative therapies. Of the nine patients who reported using cannabis for their symptoms, five reported "great improvement" in their symptoms, specifically with improvement in their mood and sleep. Two patients reported improvement in their motor symptoms and quality of life. No one reported worsening of symptoms or side effects.[9] If we can stop the negative cannabis propaganda and show patients that cannabis is like a supplement necessary for the body, patients will achieve greater control over PD symptoms and possibly slow the progression of the disease.

Jim

The first patient I observed in the dispensary with severe PD was a 70 year old gentleman named Jim. He suffered from severe rigidity, difficulty walking, slowed speech, and was unable to show expression on his face.

Jim spent his winters in Florida, and apparently some of the seniors in his area had already been using cannabis for various conditions. He had tried a few puffs off a joint several times and enjoyed the relief it provided. The biggest downside he attributed to cannabis was the offending odor since his wife would not allow him to smoke inside their home.

Jim liked the effects of inhalation and wanted to continue inhaling but wanted to use a product without the offending smell. At the time, the medical cannabis program in Connecticut did not have cannabis oil cartridges available, so I helped Jim learn how to use a Pax flower vaporizer we carried in the dispensary and sent him on his way with 1/8th of an ounce of cannabis flower.

Jim returned in under two weeks, and it was as if someone had oiled the Tin Man from "The Wizard of Oz." He was able to move his body easily and could actually show the expression on his face again. He was thrilled to be able to choose from different strains and called cannabis his most effective medication.

CBD for REM Behavioral Disturbances

One of the most destructive symptoms of severe PD is a sleep disturbance called **REM Behavior Disorder (RBD)**. RBD is characterized by a lack of muscle relaxation during REM sleep and is associated with nightmares and active behaviors during dreaming.[10] Patients can experience hallucinations while sleeping that lead to thrashing, shouting, and sometimes screaming in the middle of the night. Movements can be so severe that sleep partners have been injured when patients became violent. Clonazepam is the drug most commonly prescribed for RBD, although this class of drugs (benzodiazepines) has been linked to a worsening of dementia and should, therefore, be limited.

Patients can experience episodes of RBD *before* doctors have even made a PD diagnosis. In addition to those mentioned above, episodes can include behaviors such as laughing and singing, and patients may not remember their dreams the next morning.

A 2014 parallel, double-blind, placebo-controlled exploratory trial of CBD observed a significant reduction in RBD behavior and psychosis with doses of 75mg (3 patients) and 300mg (1 patient) of CBD per day. Patients experienced no reported side effects and when CBD was discontinued, symptoms returned.[11] This is encouraging news for patients looking for help with sleep disorders and psychosis associated with Parkinson's disease.

When treating sleep disorders with CBD, patients should medicate with cannabis throughout the day in order to balance the endocannabinoid system and take a larger dose of CBD at bedtime. If using oral products, start with 10-20mg CBD every 8 hours with a bedtime dose of 25–50mg CBD consumed 1 hour before bedtime. Increase the bedtime dose by 10mg every night until you're satisfied with the effects or, if treating multiple conditions such as pain, increase the daytime CBD dose as well.

Cannabis for "Freeze"

Patients with more advanced disease can experience medication "off" periods in which levodopa levels drop, and symptoms accelerate quickly. The "wearing-off" times can be fairly predictable, although some patients can suddenly lose the ability to move and are left helpless until more levodopa can be administered to the brain. A prescription inhaled levodopa product was recently approved by the FDA for this exact purpose.

As we have discussed, too much levodopa will cause excessive movements and can lead to hallucinations, so patients are caught between a rock and a hard place when deciding on how much levodopa to use.

Cannabis may be able to help patients relax both the mind and body and improve their motor function in times of freeze. When levodopa levels drop suddenly, patients can inhale a few puffs from a vape or place a few drops of cannabis oil under the tongue to loosen muscles and initiate movement. Products for freeze should include high amounts of both THC and CBD, although strains dominant in THC may be equally as effective.

Cannabis for Pain

Muscle rigidity and uncontrolled movements can exacerbate pain in patients with PD. As we have discussed in the chapter on pain, cannabis is effective for both muscle relaxation and nerve pain. Opioids can exacerbate confusion, hallucinations and constipation in patients with PD and are, therefore, considered a bad choice when looking for options to treat pain in patients with neurodegenerative disease. Cannabis with THC helps loosen muscle tone and decreases inflammation, which naturally leads to decreased pain. Patients can use small-inhaled doses throughout the day for mild to moderate pain or scheduled edible doses for the treatment of more severe pain or for overnight relief. (Oral doses last 6 to 12 hours.)

Orally consumed indica products for overnight relief should include CBD if patients are also experiencing other sleep issues such as REM Behavioral Disorder. CBN may offer benefits like relaxation as well, but there are no studies on the effects of CBN (cannabinol) for the treatment of Parkinson's disease. Feel free to experiment with CBN if available in your area.

Cannabis for Emotional Issues

Cannabis can help with the emotional disturbances that intensify as the disease progresses. Dopamine is linked to emotional responses, schizophrenia, and ADHD, but its exact function is not fully understood. Currently prescribed treatments for depression, specifically the drug bupropion (Wellbutrin), increase levels of dopamine in the brain since a lack of dopamine can lead to increased anxiety and depressive symptoms.

In patients with Parkinson's disease, the CB1 receptor of the endocannabinoid system has been shown to decrease expression in the substantia nigra. This effects motor, as well as emotional responses.[12, 13] Therefore, when cannabis is used properly, it can effectively treat motor and non-motor symptoms simultaneously through activation of the CB1 receptor. Anxiety and depression are a direct result of dopamine depletion from damaged neurons and a side effect of PD medications. Each additional pill can lead to more emotional side effects creating a never-ending cycle of pill after pill after pill with minimal effectiveness.

Cannabis for emotional issues should be tailored to the patient. THC offers substantial benefits for both mood and motor symptoms, so patients with mild symptoms may need a 5:1 CBD:THC ratio while patients with more advanced emotional disorders may require a 2:1 or 1:1 CBD:THC product. THC-dominant strains can offer substantial benefits on their own. Inhalation, sublingual administration, and edibles can all be of value when treating PD symptoms. Oral dosing can be administered every 6 to 12 hours for preventative care while patients with milder symptoms have the freedom to inhale from their vaporizer whenever they feel they need it. If patients experience excessive drowsiness, decrease the THC dosage by 25% or extend the dosing frequency.

A CBD-rich sativa strain that has moderate to high levels of THC will help relax patients during the day without causing excess sedation or anxiety. Indica strains can be used for relaxation at night or to help calm an aggressive patient.

Pharmacology designed to treat Parkinson's disease targets symptoms only, so choose how and when you medicate wisely. The most effective treatment for most symptoms of PD, carbidopa/levodopa, has a short window of success (around 2 years) before problems begin to arise. If patients can hold off on starting pharmaceutical medications, it will not only affect the progression of the disease but can leave more tools in the toolbox for when the disease has advanced and symptoms have become more severe.

Exercise is the only option available today that has been shown to modify disease progression.[14] Fortunately, as cannabis is decriminalized and research moves forward, we continue to discover the benefits for both treatment of underlying neurological inflammation and symptom relief. For both caregivers and the people who suffer from this brutal disease, cannabis can offer hope and comfort where there once was none.

CHAPTER 15

Cannabis and Epilepsy

"Cannabis won't kill you, but a lack of cannabinoids could."
Craig Werner[1]
Author of *Marijuana: Gateway to Health*

Epilepsy affects about fifty million people worldwide with most new cases being diagnosed in children and the elderly.[2, 3] Brain tumors, trauma, drugs, or infections in the brain can trigger abnormal seizure activity, but do not necessarily warrant a diagnosis of epilepsy.

There is not a single classification of epilepsy; there are multiple types of seizures that are categorized as either focal (occurring in one part of the brain) or generalized (occurring throughout the whole brain). Cannabis has been used to treat epileptic seizures for centuries, but only recently has real progress been made in understanding how to apply specific cannabinoids to activate the endocannabinoid receptor system in order to decrease seizure activity.

The Endocannabinoid System's Role in Epilepsy

The endocannabinoid receptor system influences seizure activity in the brain through several routes. For instance, reduced anandamide concentrations, our own naturally produced endocannabinoid, have been found in the cerebrospinal fluid of individuals with new onset temporal lobe epilepsy.[4] Endogenous cannabinoids like anandamide play a fundamental role in controlling neuronal excitability and can, therefore, open the door for the introduction of a new target for cannabinoid therapies.

Cannabis-derived cannabinoids, such as CBD and THC, are known to inhibit neurotransmitter release, but changes in receptor activity (specifically a phenomenon called "down regulation") have made applying cannabis to epileptic disorders challenging. When the right combination of cannabinoids are applied they can halt seizure activity, thereby reducing further damage to the brain from continuous, ongoing seizure activity.[5]

When using medicine to treat disease, rarely is progress a straight line. That's why medicine is considered a "practice" and not an exact science. Using cannabis to treat seizure disorders is as complicated as the underlying disease, so patients need to manage their expectations to realistic outcomes.

In this chapter, I'll help you understand the current research studies in which cannabis has successfully reduced seizure activity. I will help you learn how to begin using cannabis to reduce seizure activity, with a specific emphasis on the potential drug interactions that are possible when cannabis is combined with other anti-epileptic medications.

Patients considering cannabis for treatment of seizure disorder should seek the advice of a medical professional because drug interactions should be continually monitored through blood work, and finding the optimal combination and dosage of cannabinoids is complicated. If you have questions regarding the best way to administer your cannabis products, I am always available through my website SwayInnovations.com.

Pharmaceutical Treatments for Epilepsy: Anti-Epileptic Drugs (AEDs)

Pharmaceutical drug therapy is considered the first-line treatment for people who have had a seizure, although 3 out of 10 people taking anti-seizure medications will continue to experience seizures, leaving a window wide open to approach this problem from a different angle.[6] The goal of any treatment is to reduce seizure activity in order to slow the progression of further neuronal damage.

There are over twenty different AEDs on the market, so I won't begin to list all of the positive and negative attributes of each medication, but most carry similar side effects and frequent drug interactions. Therapies are chosen based on patient symptoms, side effect profiles, and individual patient response. Because these medications are designed to decrease over-excitability in the brain, they often do the same in the patient. Common side effects include drowsiness, fatigue, and weight gain, which can often lead to non-compliance, depression, and social isolation.

Whether a person decides to take an AED is a personal choice and should be discussed with their doctor. Although newer AED drugs have improved side effect profiles, they can still be difficult for some patients to tolerate. Anti-epileptic drugs should never be stopped suddenly or patients risk experiencing an increase in seizure activity.

AED Drug Interactions with Cannabis

Anti-epileptic drugs are known in healthcare to have frequent drug interactions. Some are minor, while others can be significant and require a change in therapy. Phenytoin, an older AED, interacts with a long list of medications and foods from over the counter omeprazole (Prilosec) to spinach. Newer drugs like levetiracetam (Keppra), a well-tolerated AED, still have a list of multiple drug interactions with normally benign drugs like Augmentin (high-dose amoxicillin).

Some of the most clinically significant drug interactions in medicine exist within the AED class. A moderate to severe drug interaction involving an AED can lead to toxic levels of one or more medications in the bloodstream, resulting in decreased respiration, liver toxicity, and excessive sedation. To avoid this, the patient's physician must continually monitor their blood work and be aware of all the drugs they are currently taking, prescription and over the counter. If abnormalities appear in the blood work, the dosages of one or more medications should be reduced or discontinued.

Drug interactions between the components of cannabis and most classes of pharmaceutical medications appear to be minimal. CBD, the molecule found to offer the most significant benefits with seizure reduction, has been shown to have some notable drug interactions detailed below. The Realm of Caring (theroc.us), a non-profit group based in Colorado that compiles current cannabis research, offers an easy-to-read chart that lists the most significant drug interactions between cannabis and pharmaceutical agents. I have summarized their chart below:

- CBD can *decrease* blood levels of clonazepam, lamotrigine, and rufinamide.
- CBD can *increase* blood levels of levetiracetam, valproate, topiramate, felbamate, and phenobarbital.

No changes in blood levels were observed when CBD was given with carbamazepine, one of the most commonly prescribed AEDs.

Below are some of the most pertinent results of studies available today regarding CBD drug interactions with AEDs:

- One study of thirteen patients with epilepsy showed that when CBD was given (initial dose 5 mg/kg/day, titrated up to a target dose of 25 mg/kg/day), a significant increase in concentrations of clobazam (Onfi, Sympazan) and its active metabolite occurred. Ten of the thirteen patients on both CBD and clobazam experienced significant side effects, and the clobazam dose had to be lowered. Clobazam is labeled for use in treating the same seizure disorders for which CBD has shown benefits.[7]
- One study showed increased levels of the active metabolites from clobazam, topiramate (Topamax), and rufinamide in both children and adults, and increased serum levels of zonisamide and eslicarbazepine in adults, as doses of CBD were increased from 5mg/kg/day to 50mg/kg/day, indicating a dose dependent interaction (the higher the dose of CBD, the greater the interaction).
- The combination of CBD and valproate may result in elevations of liver enzymes.[8]
- Carbamazepine, phenobarbital and phenytoin are known enzyme

inducers that may also increase the clearance of CBD and, therefore, reduce its availability in the bloodstream.[9] The Realm of Caring showed no interaction with carbamazepine, therefore more data is needed on this specific interaction.

This kind of information may be difficult to interpret for those not trained in pharmacology. No need to worry. The drug with the most serious drug interactions, clobazam, is a last line therapy due to serious, dangerous side effects and multiple drug interactions. The other drug interactions summarized here can be managed by your prescriber. Knowledge is power and should not be feared.

CBD Treatments for Seizure Disorders

When anti-epileptic medications fail to significantly reduce seizure activity, or patients can't tolerate their side effects, people will look for anything that may be able to help. This desperation has shown to be a catalyst in the fight to legalize cannabis as an alternative treatment for seizure disorders.

Research has found CBD to be superior to placebo for reducing the frequency of convulsive (tonic-clonic, tonic, clonic, and atonic) seizures in patients with Dravet syndrome and drop seizures in patients with Lennox-Gastaut syndrome (LGS). For the first time, there is now Class 1 evidence that suggests that the addition of CBD to current drug therapies can improve seizure control in patients with specific epilepsy syndromes.[10]

The wave of people seeking to use cannabis to treat uncontrollable seizures began with dramatic videos posted on social media showing seemingly miraculous results when children suffering from previously untreatable and uncontrollable seizure disorders stopped seizing within minutes of being given cannabis oil. A 2013 Facebook survey of parents using cannabis (35:1 CBD:THC) to treat their children who'd been diagnosed with epilepsy found an overall 84% reduction in seizures.[11]

Big numbers like these excite and offer hope to parents of children who have previously only experienced failure when using current drug therapy. But, once again, expectations for those who struggle with a seizure disorder must be realistic.

As mentioned above, CBD has been shown in clinical trials to decrease the seizure frequency in Lennox-Gastaut syndrome, a rare, severe form of epilepsy that begins in early childhood and is resistant to most anti-epileptic medications.[12] This is a fantastic discovery for parents who previously had little hope for their children who are suffering with around-the-clock seizures. Patients living with one of the many other seizure disorders may not see such dramatic results, but instead may observe smaller, more subtle benefits.

CBD may offer relief in the form of a reduction in seizure frequency, or alternatively by improving things such as alertness. Low dose CBD (10-50mg) can be stimulating for some people, while higher doses above 100mg are known to be more sedative. The current consensus is that cannabis strains high in CBD and very low in THC are most effective for seizure reduction.

There is no exact formulation of CBD and THC that works for every patient, just as there is no one pill to reduce all seizure activity in all patients. It can be frustrating for people to have to try many different drugs hoping for success, but patience when beginning cannabis therapy is required. Success has been documented with ratios of 35:1 CBD:THC and 16:1 CBD:THC, but this does not mean that other formulations somewhere in between may not work equally well.

One of my favorite articles related to cannabis use for seizure reduction was published in 2016 in *Epilepsy and Behavior*. Three physicians used cannabis to treat their patients in Washington State, California, and Maine in order to reduce seizure frequency. Patients used artisanal formulations of high CBD, low THC cannabis oil to achieve seizure reduction. Artisanal formulations are cannabis products found in cannabis dispensaries and are not approved by the FDA. (Epidiolex is an FDA-approved CBD treatment.) The following are the results the 272 combined participants from Washington and California achieved in this study:

37 (14%) found cannabis ineffective at reducing seizures.
29 (15%) experienced a 1–25% reduction in seizures.
60 (18%) experienced a 26–50% reduction in seizures.
45 (17%) experienced a 51–75% reduction in seizures.
75 (28%) experienced a 76–99% reduction in seizures.
26 (10%) experienced a complete clinical response.

"Overall, adverse effects were mild and infrequent, and beneficial side effects such as increased alertness were reported. Most patients used CBD-enriched artisanal formulas, some with the addition of Δ-9-tetra-hydrocannabinol (THC) and tetrahydrocannabinolic acid (THCA)."

Conclusions of the study:

- 21% of participants from Washington stopped taking CBD due to ineffectiveness.
- 12% of patients in California had a worsening or no relief from seizures.
- Over 1/3 of patients were able to decrease the number of anti-seizure medications, but cost was a big factor in the ability to continue treatment. Four patients experienced seizure reduction at CBD doses under 10mg per dose, substantially less expensive than doses of 100mg per dose.
- Of 272 patients, 86% had some degree of seizure reduction proving that applications for cannabis with epilepsy are promising, although "limited".
- Rescue from active seizure was helped by THC.[13]

Overall, most patients saw some seizure reduction with a substantially better side effect profile than as seen with pharmaceutical medications. As discussed earlier, drug interactions with cannabis are minor except when cannabis is used with clobazam. Although this is the case, doctors should continue to monitor blood work and patient response since clinical use of CBD is still in its early stages and we need to observe its use in larger patient populations.

Dispensary Cannabis Oil versus Pharmaceutical Products

Cannabis formulations of CBD with THC from the previous study were obtained through medical cannabis dispensaries. Inconsistency between products proved to be an issue for some of these patients. One patient saw an increase in seizure frequency when using what seemed to be an identical product to the one used earlier, but when tested showed lower levels of the terpene linalool than had been in the previous formulation. Variations between products are due to variations between plants and occur frequently in dispensaries, which can be a problem when treating patients. Standardization is required for more consistent results between oil batches.

As mentioned earlier, Epidolex is the first plant-based, FDA approved CBD formulation available in pharmacies. Studies of Epidolex include several randomized, multi-center, double-blinded, placebo-controlled trials that showed a significant reduction in seizure frequency when compared to the placebo. The most frequently reported side effects included fatigue and somnolence (drowsiness); however, diarrhea and changes in appetite were also observed. Negative side effects are often a dose-related problem. Lower doses of CBD may be as effective at reducing seizure activity as higher doses and will, more likely, have a better side effect profile. An interesting fact from the studies was that patients reported a higher overall improvement with lower doses of CBD (10 mg/kg per day) versus higher doses (20 mg/kg per day).[14] It can take some time and multiple adjustments to find your best dose of CBD with the least amount of side effects.

When comparing the study of artisanal products found in dispensaries to Epidolex, it is possible that an expanded terpene profile combined with multiple natural cannabinoids contributed to the higher success rate of the artisanal products. The relaxing terpene profile of the indica formulations seems to offer additional benefits at reducing seizure activity. This complicates the issue as terpene profiles change with each new plant grown. We want a product with a plethora of natural cannabinoids but also need some consistency between products, something that can pose a challenge in currently available treatments.

As we saw from the bell curve in Chapter 3, whole plant cannabis widen the effectiveness of the CBD molecule. The most successful case results observed in the artisanal study by Dr. Goldstein, Dr. Saneto, and Dr. Sulak was a formulation that contained CBD:CBDA:THC: THCA:THCV in a 0:7:1:6:1 ratio.[15] This shows the power of using whole plant formulations with multiple cannabinoids and the difficulty in duplicating these products at a dispensary level in order to achieve consistency between batches.

When you find an effective product for seizure reduction, list the ingredients in your journal. With today's technology in oil extraction, it is not unreasonable to expect that in the near future a manufacturer will be able to produce that exact formulation for you.

THC Use in Epilepsy and Treatment of Active Seizures

As both a proconvulsant and an anticonvulsant, using THC to treat epilepsy can be tricky. THC activity on seizure reduction appears to be dose-dependent. Low dosages of THC may help with seizure reduction while high doses of THC can cause proconvulsant activity.[16]

THC's greatest benefit for epileptic patients may be its ability to halt seizure activity when administered during an active seizure. Active seizures should be treated with sublingual oil (may be hard to administer during a seizure) or a nasal spray (rectal suppositories may work too). Stopping a seizure quickly will reduce further damage to the brain and can save a person's life.

Pharmacology to halt an active seizure consists of a group of medicines called benzodiazepines; diazepam [Diastat rectal gel, lorazepam

(Ativan), and midazolam (Versed)]. It can only benefit patients to have additional safe and effective rescue medications that are easily administered available. Cannabis products for administration during a seizure are nasal, rectal, or possibly buccal (those you can rub into a cheek).

Nasal Spray Rescue from Cannatol Rx is a 1:20 CBD:THC spray that can stop a seizure in seconds when 5mg of THC is administered up the nose.

Although effective as a rescue remedy, if THC is regularly smoked in high amounts or consumed as a high-dose edible, THC blood levels can reduce the seizure threshold resulting in an uptick in seizure activity.

I witnessed the effects THC can have on seizure frequency when Becky, a thirty-three-year-old female cerebral palsy patient, came into the dispensary looking for help to reduce her daily onslaught of seizures.

Becky

Becky was born with cerebral palsy. Her mom, Susie, told me she had been experiencing multiple seizures every day since she was born. When she arrived with her mom for a consultation, Becky was unable to speak and was using a wheelchair because the never-ending seizures she experienced inflicted significant damage to her brain. She had the intellectual capabilities of a small child and required around the clock care, which Susie and her husband provided.

Susie was hopeful that CBD could reduce Becky's seizures and help with some aggressive behavior issues Becky had during the day.

Becky started on a solution of cannabis oil dissolved in MCT oil that contained high amounts of CBD combined with almost no THC. Her mother saw an immediate improvement in the number of seizures Becky had per day. Unfortunately, Becky's parents also saw an uptick in her aggressive behavior and emotional outbursts every afternoon around 2:00 p.m. that would last for hours. When searching for a more relaxing product with the ability to control seizures, we found one that contained high amounts of CBN (cannabinol) combined with very low amounts of THC. CBN is derived from the THC molecule but has very little psychoactive effects and is thought to be relaxing.

Susie gave Becky a small dose of CBN at noon and a higher dose 1 hour before bedtime in order to, hopefully, enable Becky to sleep past 5:00 a.m., a huge benefit for Susie and her husband. The CBN worked well to control Becky's aggressive afternoon behavior and helped her sleep later into the mornings (thus making Susie a happier mama).

After about three months, we ran into a common problem within the cannabis industry, a lack of product availability. Becky's CBN oil supply had run out, and the manufacturer of the product needed at least three to six months to replenish their supply.

In the meantime, we decided to try a small dose of an indica-based THC product in place of the CBN to help relax Becky and reduce her aggressive behaviors. I told Susie to stop giving Becky the THC cookie if she noticed any increase in Becky's seizure activity.

At first, the switch to the indica-based THC product seemed to solve the problem. The seizures did not increase in frequency, and Becky was happier and more relaxed. But after a couple of months, Susie told me that Becky was having more seizures.

I asked Susie to document every dose of every medication given to Becky over a 48-hour period. Once analyzed, I discovered that somehow Becky was now taking more THC throughout the day than CBD. Because the THC products had improved Becky's behavior, I assumed that her parents had just started to give her a little bit more over time until the THC had become a pro-convulsant and seizure frequency once again began to increase.

I was correct. Once we discovered the problem, we were able to return to the original dosing pattern of high CBD with lower THC and, once again, the seizures decreased in frequency.

THCA Treatment for Seizure Disorders

THCA (tetrahydrocannabinolic acid) is the acid form of the active THC molecule that is abundant in the raw plant before decarboxylation. THCA does not exhibit the psychotropic side effects associated with THC, but may produce beneficial anticonvulsant effects and can be used in combination with CBD, or alone for patients for whom CBD is not effective (which can be up to 20% of patients).

Dr. Bonni Goldstein and Dr. Dustin Sulak wrote about their use of THCA when treating epileptic seizures, and how they found success using very small doses: 0.01–2 mg/kg/day THCA with or without additional CBD.[16] Greater efficacy was not seen in higher doses. They saw the greatest benefit when patients took a combination of CBD, CBDA, THC, THCA and THCV. (THCV is a cannabinoid that is being looked at for its benefits in seizure reduction.)

If you have access to THCA, either use it alone at very low doses (1-2mg every 8 hours) or combine it with CBD to see if it will offer additional benefits.

Beginning CBD Therapy

In Chapter 3 you learned about the importance of locating the sweet spot when dosing CBD. High doses of CBD can be as ineffective as low doses of CBD and can result in increased sedation and other negative side effects. CBD's effectiveness follows a bell curve and must be tailored to the individual patient. Over the counter CBD products can be used for seizure reduction, but they often do not contain additional terpenes that may affect the results.

When beginning CBD therapy (with or without THC) dosages should be initiated at low levels and slowly increased until optimal effects are observed. For some patients, a 25–50% reduction in seizures is the maximum benefit CBD can offer (still pretty good).

It is natural that most patients will continue to increase their CBD dosage to see if more positive outcomes are observed at higher and higher doses. If you continue to increase the dosage of CBD and do not observe additional benefits (or negative side effects develop), then you should decrease the dosage until the negative side effects subside while still maintaining optimal benefits with seizure frequency.

This can best be accomplished by using your journal. Each day write down the time and dosage given along with seizure frequency. Over time you will be able to determine the dosage that corresponds to the least amount of seizures. If you have trouble interpreting the data, please contact me at SwayInnovations.com for a consultation. Lower doses will equate to significant cost savings as well as reduced side effects.

When I started working with epileptic patients in the dispensary, Epidiolex was not available. I based my recommended dosages for patients on the information provided at the Realm of Caring. Today Epidiolex begins their dosing at 2.5mg/kg/day increasing up to 20mg/kg/day.[17] The Realm of Caring has a Pediatric Cannabinoid Dosing Guideline that begins at 0.5mg/kg/day (0.25mg/kg/day for drug-sensitive patients) in two to three divided doses.[18] I believe that starting with lower dosages, like those provided by Realm of Caring, is better than starting at higher dosages.

How to Determine Optimal Daily Dosage of CBD

To determine your daily dose of CBD, you must first convert your weight into kilograms (kg). Divide your weight in pounds (lb.) by 2.2. Then multiply this number by 0.5mg (for a starting dose), and you'll have the amount that needs to be given over the entire day. Divide this amount by the number of doses to be given per day and that's it.

> **For example, a 50lb. patient would have a calculation like this:**
> 50lb./2.2 = 22.7kg x 0.5mg/day starting dose = 11.4mg per day
> 11.4 divided by 3 (doses every 8 hours) gives
> an approximate starting dose of 4mg every
> 8 hours or 6mg every 12 hours.

Patients should remain on a dose for five to seven days to observe the effects completely before increasing the dosage. The dosage can be slowly increased every week until negative side effects appear or benefits decrease.

If all this seems too confusing, I created a simple dosing schedule to help you get started (see below). For small children, it is best to use the more precise weight-based formula, but this chart may be easier to follow when applied to adults. Some patients better tolerate medications when lower doses are given more frequently, so if you find higher over-all dosages are more effective in controlling seizure frequency but give unpleasant side effects, consider smaller amounts dosed every 6 hours instead of higher doses every 12 hours.

Initiating CBD Therapy (simple method):

2mg CBD every 12 hours x 5 days

5mg CBD every 12 hours x 1 week

10mg CBD every 12 hours x 1 week

15mg CBD every 12 hours x 1 week

20mg CBD every 12 hours x 1 week

(Add 5mg of CBD to each dose every week.)

If seizure activity increases, the dosages should be decreased until you once again see improvement. For patients with regular seizure activity, do not suddenly stop a high dose CBD treatment, because this may exacerbate seizure activity. Instead, reduce the dose slowly every 5 days over the course of 3 to 4 weeks or speak with your prescriber.

There is a lot to consider when initiating cannabinoid therapy, including the risks, benefits, and significant costs for all anti-seizure medications. Patients can face compelling challenges when accessing cannabis preparations, including high costs and a lack of consistency between available products. Patients in the 2016 Washington and California study frequently followed low sugar, low carbohydrate diets in addition to using cannabis products. One of the most successful cases observed in the ongoing Washington and California study is a combination of five cannabinoids (CBD, CBDA, THC, THCA and CBN). This demonstrates that lower doses of multiple cannabinoids consumed together may offer improved results over higher doses of a single cannabinoid.

One important aspect of cannabis that seems to effect seizure frequency is the use of an indica strain versus a sativa strain. Indica strains have higher concentrations of terpenes such as myrcene and linalool. These molecules provide relaxing effects, which may help decrease the excitability of the epileptic brain. The terpenes of indica strains seem to have beneficial additive effects to dispensary formulations.

Although cannabis has been used for centuries to reduce seizure frequency, we are just beginning to understand how to apply whole-plant products consistently to all epileptic patients, a daunting task. The more we learn, the more hope can be offered to patients who experience uncontrollable seizure activity.

420: code for cannabis smoke time (4:20), or referring to April 20th (4/20) which is considered the national holiday for cannabis culture.

CHAPTER 16

Mental Health with a Focus on Anxiety and Depression

*"The illegality of cannabis is outrageous, an impediment
to full utilization of a drug which helps produce the serenity
and insight, sensitivity and fellowship so desperately needed
in this increasingly mad and dangerous world."*
Carl Sagan[1]

Mental and emotional afflictions range from occasional nervousness and anxiety to deep, dark depression accompanied by a complete withdrawal from society. People with deep, emotional pain may find it difficult to get the kind of help they need, whether it be a lack of available services, intolerable or expensive medications, or an inability to reach out for help. Mental health services in the United States are almost an afterthought in healthcare, oftentimes barely covered by insurance, when mental stability is the cornerstone of a productive, successful citizen. For those that do seek help, answers doled out in pills offer erratic and inconsistent success. Some people do well with currently available antidepressants, while others continue to suffer. Self-medication comes in the form of alcohol, sex, food—anything that is easily accessible and can numb the pain becomes the prescription by which many choose to abide.

Anxiety disorders affect about forty million adults aged eighteen and older in the United States and are our most common mental health issue.[2] These numbers are staggering, yet they may be even higher since many people with mental health issues do not seek treatment because of a sense of shame regarding their condition. It is not an understatement to say this is a complex problem.

In this chapter, I focus on cannabis use for anxiety and depression. Pharmacology for these issues focuses treatment on the neurotransmitters serotonin, norepinephrine, dopamine, but the effectiveness of these drugs is, shall we say, underwhelming. Studies have shown some of the functions of the endocannabinoid system are to influence our fear response, acute and long-term depression, and anxiety, making the ERS a suitable target for additional treatments.

Dr. Amy Barnhorst is a psychiatrist who recently wrote an article for the *New York Times* called "The Empty Promise of Suicide Prevention" in which she reports that only 40–60% of patients who take antidepressants actually feel better. This means roughly half of people seeking insurance-sanctioned medication for mood disorders will find the available drugs inadequate. Nearly one in ten Americans are on an antidepressant, yet there is little convincing evidence they actually reduce suicides.[3] As a cruel twist of fate, most antidepressants contain a black box warning where the use of these medications may increase the risk of suicide, especially in the first few weeks after starting therapy.

Pharmaceutical Treatments for Anxiety and Depression

There are four classes of drugs that are currently considered first-line treatments for the majority of depressive disorders in the United States (with specific exceptions, of course). I will not be discussing drugs used for atypical depression, such as antipsychotic medications. Drugs used to treat anxiety and depression focus on increasing the neurotransmitters serotonin, norepinephrine, and/or dopamine.

The first drugs to be used as antidepressants, MAO inhibitors and tricyclic antidepressants, were introduced in the 1950s, but these came with significant and sometimes deadly side effects.[4] Their use has waned in recent decades.

Prozac, the first selective serotonin re-uptake inhibitor (SSRI) to come to market in 1987, burst on the scene as the miracle drug society needed to combat the stressors of life.[5] Although some patients find relief with pharmaceuticals, others can experience negative side effects including suicidal thoughts or a worsening of their depressive symptoms. Thirty years after Prozac's arrival, the limitations of these medications have become increasingly evident and new therapeutic targets are needed.

Below is a list of the most commonly prescribed classes of drugs used to treat mood disorders:

SSRI: Selective Serotonin Re-uptake Inhibitors were the first drugs to focus on the serotonin receptor system to treat depression, specifically a receptor known as 5-HT_{1A}. SSRIs include drugs like fluoxetine (Prozac), sertraline (Zoloft), citalopram (Celexa), and escitalopram (Lexapro).

SNRI: Serotonin Norepinephrine Re-uptake Inhibitors increase serotonin in the brain along with norepinephrine. Some of these medications have been approved for chronic pain as well as depression. SNRIs include duloxetine (Cymbalta) and venlafaxine (Effexor).

NDRI: Norepinephrine-Dopamine Re-uptake Inhibitors increase the amount of norepinephrine and dopamine in the brain. Included in this class is the popular drug bupropion (Wellbutrin, Zyban), which has been used for depression, weight loss, and smoking cessation.

Tricyclic Antidepressants: Like SNRIs, tricyclics increase the amount of serotonin and norepinephrine in the brain, as well as another neurotransmitter, acetylcholine. Increasing acetylcholine has led to negative cardiac side effects resulting in a decline in prescribing rates in recent years.

When comparing available antidepressants, most show similar efficacy for treating depression, although side effects differ between drugs and drug classes.[6] With a sole focus on the serotonin, norepinephrine, and dopamine neurotransmitters, it seems as if each new drug that is introduced to the market brings few new benefits other than a different set of side effects.

A recent article on InformedHealth.org compared how ineffective antidepressants were at treating symptoms in adults with moderate to severe depression. The results are compelling:

Without antidepressants, 20 to 40 people out of one hundred (20–40%) who took a placebo noticed an improvement in their symptoms within six to eight weeks.

With antidepressants, 40 to 60 people out of one hundred (40–60%) who took an antidepressant noticed an improvement in their symptoms within six to eight weeks.

In other words, antidepressants improved symptoms in just twenty additional people out of one hundred (20%) when compared to a patient taking nothing (placebo).[7] That leaves a large group of people living with unsatisfactory results.

Recently, it came to light how difficult and dangerous it can be for patients to stop using antidepressants when they no longer feel they need them. I know patients that refused to start using an antidepressant for fear they would have to take it for the rest of their life. As a pharmacist working in a community pharmacy, I witnessed how difficult it was for patients to stop taking their antidepressants. Every weekend, patients came to the pharmacy desperate to get a few pills to hold them over until they could get a refill from their doctor on Monday. These people made the mistake of thinking they could just stop taking their antidepressant for a few days, but quickly realized they could not stop taking their medication voluntarily. For many patients, the inability to stop using their antidepressant was a wakeup call that was extremely upsetting.

A new approach to treating major depression has recently been introduced with the expanded use of ketamine, a drug that induces a state of dissociative anesthesia to rapidly reduce suicidal thoughts and other serious symptoms of depression. Ketamine has an interesting history in medicine since its introduction in 1970.[8] It has mainly been used to induce sedation during surgery, but also happens to be in the class of drugs used to treat Alzheimer's disease, NMDA receptor antagonists, the most famous of which is memantine (Namenda). Ketamine has shown great promise in treating major depression symptoms for patients that do not respond to first-line medications like SSRIs and SNRIs.

Problems with Benzodiazepines or "Benzos"

Antidepressant medications are prescribed for both depression and generalized anxiety disorders. A daily antidepressant is considered a preventative approach when treating anxiety while a class of drugs called benzodiazepines, or "benzos," are used to treat acute anxiety symptoms. The most common benzodiazepines prescribed for anxiety are lorazepam (Ativan), clonazepam (Klonopin) diazepam (Valium), and alprazolam (Xanax).

Benzodiazepines have been widely prescribed for sleep and anxiety, but a recent study revealed a link between benzodiazepines and an increased risk of Alzheimer's disease.[9] Benzodiazepines are associated with abuse and dependency issues, a problem seen daily in pharmacy practice. High doses of a benzodiazepine can actually make anxiety worse, so patients can find themselves stuck in a spin cycle where they feel anxious, take a pill, then when the effects of that pill wear off, they feel more anxious, so they take another pill and so on and so on. What was prescribed to relieve anxiety becomes the source of their anxiety when taken at higher and higher dosages.

Benzodiazepines are administered with a warning that they may cause dependency, but antidepressants are not listed as a controlled medication, and, therefore, do not warn patients of the complications they may encounter when trying to stop using them for treatment. Perhaps cannabis can offer an alternative to this pharmaceutical ball and chain.

Cannabis Treatments for Anxiety and Depression

When cannabis is used to treat anxiety and depression, just like all medications, it can take a little time to find the right fit. CBD, with its lack of euphoria, is the milder of the two cannabinoids and ideal for patients who want to begin cannabis therapy but feel a bit nervous about sampling THC. If CBD is too mild, low-dose THC can be added for increased relaxation. I found that for most patients a combination of cannabinoids is most effective.

Terpenes add beneficial, synergistic significance to cannabinoid action and particular attention should be paid to strains for daytime use. Very relaxing strains used during the day can exacerbate symptoms of depression and cause excessive sedation in some patients while a strong sativa strain can increase anxiety in sensitive patients. The right hybrid, combining THC and CBD, can most often be the perfect fit.

Best Cannabis for Treating Anxiety

Without a doubt, cannabis can be used to replace your benzodiazepine medications, such as alprazolam (Xanax) or lorazepam (Ativan), no matter how high your dosage. The group that receives the most benefit from removing benzodiazepines from their drug regimen is the group to whom it is most often prescribed, senior patients. Seniors are frequently prescribed benzodiazepines for anxiety even though these drugs carry an increased risk of Alzheimer's disease. It's imperative that we use a better option, like cannabis. Cannabinoids can work as an alternative to benzodiazepines to relieve anxiety, with the added benefits of providing additional pain relief and a reduction of chronic inflammation. That sounds like a dream drug for everybody!

Many people are skeptical about cannabis' ability to help them stop using their benzodiazepines without experiencing more anxiety, but everyone I observed who has wanted to stop (no matter how high the dose) was able to stop without experiencing increased anxiety or withdrawal symptoms after they found the right cannabis product. It may sound miraculous, but it is reality. I have witnessed it again and again with people who laughed at me when I told them it was possible. Patients often worry that they will go through withdrawal if they "can't have" their next anxiety pill. I tell them to keep taking their pills as prescribed and once they find the right cannabis product at the right dose, they just won't need that next pill. Speak with your prescriber about a taper schedule to help slowly remove or reduce your current benzodiazepine usage.

Studies show CBD to be effective for treating mild to moderate anxiety.[10] For patients new to the world of medical cannabis, CBD is often the perfect entry point because it doesn't come with psychoactive side effects. It is very mild and, if not strong enough, can be combined with other cannabinoids like CBN or THC for a totally different experience. Refer to Chapter 3 for how to effectively begin using CBD.

In my experience, ideal strains for anxiety are rich in CBD and have low to moderate amounts of THC and a relaxing terpene profile. For mild to moderate anxiety, a 5:1 ratio of CBD:THC can work well, while more severe anxiety can be treated with a 3:1 or 2:1 CBD:THC product. High CBD blends are often marketed for pain, but they are also excellent for treating anxiety.

While low doses of THC can help decrease anxiety, high dosages can absolutely increase anxiety symptoms. If you notice your anxiety increasing as you begin using cannabis, consider changing strains or lowering your THC doses.

Avoid strong, full sativa strains if you deal with anxiety. Sativa-dominant hybrids (sativa crossed with an indica) are still wakeful and non-drowsy but less likely to cause anxiety than full sativa strains. These strains (Jack Herrer and Blue Dream) can be perfect for daytime use.

A full, balanced hybrid will offer more relaxation than a sativa strain, but some people find themselves drowsy later in the day. If this happens to you, reduce your dosage (high-dose THC can cause drowsiness), increase the amount of CBD in your product, or try a more sativa-dominant strain.

Some patients prefer to inhale whenever they feel anxious while others with more chronic symptoms prefer the long, relaxing effects provided by consuming cannabis as an edible. If your anxiety seems to be getting worse, consider decreasing the amount of THC you're using and increase the levels of CBD. Make sure you are not using a sativa formulation, but rather an indica-based CBD strain which can be relaxing without being heavily sedating.

The goal is a balance of cannabinoids and terpenes that relaxes you without causing drowsiness.

Quick Tips when Choosing Products for Anxiety:

1. Begin with a CBD-rich product that has little to no THC. If purchasing from a dispensary, use an indica-based CBD product for anxiety. If purchasing CBD oil from a store, see if they offer samples. I have found some great products in the CBD stores popping up all over my hometown. A good quality CBD product found online is called Hemp Gummies (www.TribeCBD.com).

2. If CBD is not effective, consider adding THC in a 5:1, 3:1 or 2:1 CBD:THC ratio. These products can be inhaled to quickly decrease anxiety symptoms. Choose strains with a relaxing terpene profile, if possible. If consumed as an edible, consider a starting dose of 10mg CBD with 2-3mg THC.

3. If using THC dominant strains, avoid full sativa strains initially. If you're looking for a daytime product that contains THC, use sativa-dominant hybrids or full hybrids. Indica strains are used during the day by patients with severe anxiety, but most patients find them too sedating to use continually throughout the day.

A Layered Approach to Treating Anxiety

If you live with a chaotic mind, racing thoughts, and tightness in the chest and throat, cannabis may be able to offer some relief. As someone who lives with anxiety myself, and has helped hundreds of people find the right products to treat their own anxiety, I know that cannabis can be one of the best tools in the toolbox for those of us living with bouts of anxiety. *But,* it is not a cure.

Anxiety is a symptom of an overactive nervous system and must be treated accordingly. In order to work best, cannabis should be part of a multi-faceted approach to helping the body and mind reduce symptoms of stress and regain a sense of peace and calm.

Quick-Tips to Reduce Anxiety without Medication:

1. Reduce or eliminate caffeine. It is a stimulant that contributes to anxiety. You'll probably say it does not affect your anxiety, but I promise, caffeine is a strong drug that does contribute to anxiety symptoms.

2. Clean up your diet. Do you eat a lot of sugary, processed foods? Again, these are stimulants to the nervous system. More and more studies support how powerful and destructive sugar can be to the body and mind.

3. Exercise exhausts the body to release toxic thoughts. Yoga is both meditative and exhaustive, but vigorous exercise can work just as well at calming the anxious mind. Burn it off!

4. Meditate. Meditation has been shown to produce physiological changes in a person's body by decreasing cortisol and increasing immunoglobulin A, our body's natural defense against bacteria and viruses. Most people like the idea of meditation but don't know how to do it. Be easy on yourself and give it a try. Meditation is *extremely* effective for anxiety and, best of all, is free! I prefer not to meditate in silence and use a free app called Mindstate. Headspace is also a free app and helpful for beginners. The purpose of meditation is to calm your mind and choose your thoughts like you choose your clothes every day. To let the mind roam free without restriction can put people with depression and anxiety in a very dark place. For some reason, the mind will automatically create a

---

negative future outcome (usually it never comes to fruition) or reaches back to painful, past experiences. Either way, it removes the joy from the present moment. The only goal with meditation is to keep doing it every day. It is a skill that can be strengthened and, dare I say, nothing is more effective for an anxious mind. It is that powerful.

Best Cannabis for Depression

Patients take antidepressants for all kinds of reasons. Life is brutal, sometimes overwhelming, and an antidepressant can help level out erratic emotions, which can cause problems in a marriage or a job. If you have moved through a difficult time in your life and are ready to stop taking your antidepressant, I strongly advise having a conversation with your doctor about your goals. Your doctor should listen to your concerns, help to decide if removing the medication is a good idea, develop a tapering schedule, monitor your progress and offer supportive care. No one should attempt to stop an antidepressant without support. Emotional and physical side effects can be extreme, so be kind to your body. Take it slow.

The most widely prescribed antidepressants are completely out of your system in about a week (Lexapro, 7 days; Zoloft, 6 days; and Celexa, 8 days), but it can take months for your brain chemistry to re-adjust to living without these medications. This can be challenging. Cannabis can help relieve anxiety symptoms of withdrawal, sleep disturbances, and muscle tightness while helping directly with depression in its own right.

Start with CBD

Scientific evidence is mounting in support of the antidepressant effects of CBD, not necessarily through the endocannabinoid receptor system, but through a different receptor we are already familiar with in depression, the serotonin receptor 5-HT_{1A}. In addition, a biomarker called brain-derived neurotrophic factor (BDNF) has been shown to be deplet-ed in patients with depression and was shown to be elevated in animals who were given CBD.[11]

When starting cannabis for depression, the lack of euphoric effects associated with CBD makes it the easier molecule to tolerate for most people, although we don't want to discount the benefits THC provides for depression. If using a hemp-derived CBD product (sold over the counter or online), look for products marketed for daytime use that con-tain multiple cannabinoids. Hemp or dispensary products containing sativa terpenes, such as limonene, will help depressive symptoms better than products that are more sedating. (Sedating products can be used for sleep or anxiety). I recently tried a CBD oil sold at a store in town and found it very relaxing. It was a combination of CBD, CBG, CBN, and CBDV, but did not contain additional terpenes.

Refer to Chapter 3 to learn how to effectively dose CBD. The most common side effects resulting from CBD use are headache, upset stom-ach, and sedation. These tend to appear at higher doses, so if you begin to develop negative side effects, decrease your daily dosage by 25%. It can take 4-6 weeks for antidepressants to become fully effective. This may also be true when using CBD for depression. Once you have taken dosages of 25–100mg CBD per day with no observable benefits, it may be time to add some uplifting THC (2–5mg).

Adding THC

If relief from CBD is inadequate, the next step is to use THC alone or in combination with CBD to decrease THC-induced euphoria. THC has shown to have antidepressant effects when given to mice, and I have wit-nessed patients who experienced seemingly miraculous results from the use of sativa THC products in the dispensary setting.[12] One patient with lifelong, intractable depression found relief with 10mg of a sativa edible taken twice a day (every 6 to 8 hours), while another patient with a very high tolerance took 100mg once a day in the morning and said it was the best antidepressant he had ever taken in his life. If treating depression combined with anxiety, I would highly recommend beginning with a combination of THC and CBD. If you suffer from depression without anxiety, you may do better with sativa THC and little CBD. There is no wrong place to begin, it's wherever you feel most comfortable.

To start using THC for depression, combine 10–20mg of CBD with 2–5mg of THC. For those who prefer inhaled products, look for sativa strains rich in CBD. Remember, sativa for daytime and indica at night. Sativa THC products elevate mood but can cause sedation when the THC dose is too high. So, if you are drowsy during the day, consider decreasing your dosage by 25%. As stated in Chapter 3, do not re-medicate with an edible for 6 hours, otherwise, you won't be able to evaluate the dose completely. Write the dose and results in your journal. If you felt the effects were too weak, keep the CBD at 20-30mg and increase your THC dose by 2–5mg every other day until you're satisfied. If you increase your dose too quickly you may find it hard to "dial-in" your best dosage. Listen to your body and take your time. If something does not feel good, make adjustments. More cannabis is not better; it's just more likely to cause negative side effects, so listen to your body and take it slow.

As mentioned previously, using a product (inhaled or edible) that contains more CBD than THC will decrease the euphoria associated with THC. This may be preferable during working hours, so experiment with different strains and products. Less euphoria can also equate to less anxiety.

CHAPTER 17

Gastrointestinal (GI) Disorders

"We have been terribly and systematically misled
[regarding marijuana] for nearly 70 years in the United States,
and I apologize for my own role in that."
Dr. Sanjay Gupta[1]
CNN.com Chief Medical Correspondent

Gastrointestinal disorders include dozens of diagnoses from heartburn to cancer and stretch from the esophagus through thirty feet of gastrointestinal tract ending at the rectum. There are sixty to seventy million people affected by GI disorders, and almost a quarter of a million people die every year as a direct result.[2,3] Fear, depression, and anxiety develop as patients must navigate food like a minefield. Pharmacology for conditions of the GI tract include some of the most profitable drugs in the world, drugs like Humira and Enbrel, which are approved for moderate to severe inflammatory diseases like Crohn's disease and Ulcerative colitis, and produce around nine billion dollars *each* in sales every year. These highly profitable medications come with more than a high sticker price. Each drug includes a list of severe, even life-threatening side effects, three of which are listed as black box warnings, the strictest labeling requirements required by the FDA. Most drugs that list a black box warning only list one.

It should come as no surprise that Big Pharma continues to fight hard to keep cannabis illegal. The anti-inflammatory actions of cannabis coupled with a lower cost and better safety profile will cost the pharmaceutical industry billions upon billions of dollars in lost profits. But it's only a matter of time before cannabis takes its rightful place as an effective, mainstream, alternative medication.

The endocannabinoid receptor system plays a significant role in the health and comfort of our GI tract, yet no drug besides dronabinol (a synthetic THC molecule marketed before the endocannabinoid system was even discovered thirty years ago) targets treatment on this particular receptor system. CB2 receptors are present throughout the GI tract and affect motility, inflammation, and hunger signaling.[4] According to researchers at the University of Naples Federico II, cannabinoids "provide a new therapeutic target for the treatment of a number of gastrointestinal diseases, including nausea and vomiting, gastric ulcers, secretory diarrhea, paralytic ileus, inflammatory bowel disease, colon cancer, and gastro-esophageal reflux conditions."[5]

It is time to validate cannabis as an effective medicine for GI disorders, and approach the endocannabinoid receptor system as a new therapeutic target for treatment of GI disease. This chapter summarizes medications commonly used for GI issues and focuses on how to use cannabis to decrease inflammation and calm the most common symptoms associated with gastrointestinal disease.

Pharmaceutical Treatments for Gastrointestinal Disorders

Pharmaceutical drugs often have a single labeled indication, which directs their effects like a missile to a target. This approach may be appropriate when treating infections with an antibiotic but falls short when dealing with an organ system as large, complex, and intricate as the gastrointestinal tract. Most GI drugs are designed to decrease the body's natural immune response leading to unintended negative consequences like secondary infections and cancer. Below are the most prevalent therapies prescribed for the most common problems of the GI tract and the negative side effects associated with these medications:

TNF antagonists include drugs such as infliximab (Remicade), adalimumab (Humira), and etanercept (Enbrel), which are used to treat moderate to severe inflammatory conditions such as rheumatoid arthritis, psoriasis, Crohn's disease (CD) and Ulcerative colitis (UC). They non-selectively block an inflammatory cytokine, Tumor Necrosis Factor (TNF), which suppresses the entire body's natural immune system leading to a host of serious side effects. All five TNF antagonists have been issued not one, but three black box warnings, assigned in 2008, 2009 and a third in 2011. They include:

- increased risk for developing serious infections including tuberculosis (TB), histoplasmosis, listeriosis, and Pneumocystis (pneumonia) that may lead to hospitalization or death (2008)
- increased risk of developing lymphoma and other malignancies, some fatal, in children and adolescent patients (2009)
- post-marketing cases of fatal hepatosplenic T-cell lymphoma (HSTCL), a rare type of T-cell lymphoma (2011)[6]

Anti-nausea medications, such as ondansetron (Zofran) and prochlorperazine (Compazine), can be extremely effective at reducing nausea but do not increase appetite like cannabis can. Prochlorperazine contains a black box warning prohibiting its use in patients with dementia. Ondansetron (Zofran) is widely prescribed but can lead to a serious side effect called serotonin syndrome as well as cardiac irregularities, fatigue, urinary retention, and constipation.

Corticosteroids, such as prednisone and dexamethasone, have been used to decrease inflammation for over seventy-five years. They are extremely effective for rheumatoid arthritis, cancer, and multiple sclerosis, but long-term use comes with a long list of severe side effects. They are not, therefore, to be considered acceptable therapy for chronic inflammation. Long-term steroid use can lead to changes in the face (called a Cushingoid appearance), weight gain, high blood pressure, immunosuppression, pancreatitis, glaucoma, osteoporosis, and growth suppression.

Metoclopramide is the only drug still available in the drug class of pro-kinetics since cisapride (Propulsid) was removed from the market in

2000 due to heart rhythm deaths.[7] Metoclopramide is widely prescribed to increase the motility of the GI tract for treating conditions such as nausea and heartburn. Although frequently used, most patients would be surprised to know that metoclopramide has a black box warning regarding the possibility of developing an irreversible movement disorder, called tardive dyskinesia, which is normally associated with antipsychotic drugs. In 2017, the FDA approved two drugs for treatment of the tardive dyskinesia, valbenazine (Ingrezza) and deutetrabenazine (Austedo).[8] Metoclopramide has also been linked to Parkinson's-like syndrome, seizures, and severe cardiac irregularities.

Cytoprotectant agents, such as misoprostol, stimulate blood flow through the lining of the GI tract and increase mucus production. This forms a protective layer when treating gastric ulcers. Once again, misoprostol contains a black box warning to limit treatment to less than twelve weeks to reduce the risk of forming tardive dyskinesia. Misoprostol can cause birth defects, high blood pressure, and severe cardiac issues.

Aminosalicylates are a class of drugs that include mesalamine, an anti-inflammatory molecule, to treat chronic inflammation associated with Crohn's disease (CD) and Ulcerative colitis (UC). According to Cochrane.org, ten studies concluded that sulfasalazine, the most widely prescribed oral drug in the aminosalicylates class, is only moderately effective for the treatment of active Crohn's disease, and mesalamine shows limited benefit.[9] The side effects, as usual, are expansive and severe: liver toxicity, kidney toxicity, and infertility are on the list.

Thiopurines work to suppress the body's natural immune system similar to the way TNF antagonists work but through a different pathway. Azathioprine and its active metabolite, mercaptopurine, are widely prescribed to reduce inflammation from active disease. Tioguanine was originally used to treat leukemia and as an alternative for patients who could not tolerate azathioprine and mercaptopurine. They have been shown to be effective for promoting remission during active disease, but all three drugs carry a significant risk of liver toxicity as well as secondary cancers due to suppression of immune functions.[10]

Antispasmodics relax the smooth muscle of the intestinal wall to reduce spasms due to Irritable Bowel Syndrome (IBS). The most commonly prescribed medication for IBS is dicyclomine, a drug that works by blocking acetylcholine. Drugs used to treat dementia aim to increase the amount of acetylcholine in the brain, so you can see how a problem may develop when using these two medications simultaneously. Side effects of dicyclomine are mild, but so are the results. Many, many people find it to be ineffective for relieving severe GI discomfort.

I like to summarize the medications used for GI disorders so you can see the level of toxicity associated with the pharmaceutical treatments for chronic inflammatory bowel conditions. Many of these drugs lower the body's natural immune response, which can be dangerous as it can lead to the development of cancer and serious secondary infections. If we can significantly reduce the dosages of these medications by adding cannabis to the treatment regimens, it is possible patients could have a better response with less toxic side effects.

GI disorders are chronic conditions that require ongoing treatment, and most of these medications have side effects that worsen dramatically as patients remain on the drug. As evidence continues to accumulate, cannabis should and will be offered as a first-line treatment for all gastrointestinal disorders instead of only being available or recommended as a last option.

Cannabis Treatments for Gastrointestinal Disorders

The endocannabinoid receptor system is found throughout the gastrointestinal tract and offers a new therapeutic target for GI disorders. To oversimplify cannabinoid applications, CBD is used for inflammation and THC is used for spasms, nausea, vomiting and to increase the appetite. Refer to Chapter 2 for a full list of applications for each cannabinoid. Inhaled products are ideal for acute symptoms, while oral products may offer a better approach for the prevention of chronic symptoms. Micro-dosing, as discussed in Chapter 3, could also be an effective dosing technique for chronic GI conditions. Below I talk about the most common symptoms associated with gastrointestinal disease and how to use cannabis to treat them. Please refer to Chapter 8 for instruction on how to specifically treat pain.

Inflammation and Spasms

As we have discussed throughout this book, inflammation is a significant underlying contributor to the most severe and chronic diseases of the human body. Inflammatory Bowel Disease (IBD), which includes Crohn's disease (CD) and Ulcerative colitis (UC), is characterized by chronic, relapsing inflammatory episodes that cause loose stools, bleeding, malabsorption, and abdominal pain. In Israel, cannabis has been legally registered as a palliative treatment for both CD and UC[11]

The synergy between THC and CBD for the treatment of stomach discomfort is well documented scientifically and understood through anecdotal evidence. As previously discussed, CBD is a potent anti-inflammatory and antioxidant—exactly what is required to effectively treat inflammatory conditions of the bowel. Both THC and CBD have anti-inflammatory properties and have been shown to improve colitis in rodents.[12, 13]

Treating inflammation can require high levels of CBD with lower amounts of THC, although we must not forget that THC is anti-inflammatory in its own right and may be preferable for some people. Refer to Chapter 3 for how to effectively use CBD orally. Since THC also works to decrease inflammation and spasms, a combination of equal parts CBD and THC is a great place to start when treating inflammation and to combat active symptoms.

For spasm relief, THC is the more effective cannabinoid. However, products that combine both THC and CBD may feel more comfortable mentally for patients, especially during working hours. Patients sensitive to THC should begin with CBD-rich strains with lower levels of THC such as a 4:1 or 3:1 CBD:THC ratio. The amount of THC required will be patient-specific. Severe pain and spasms may require higher doses of THC, so consider products with a 2:1 or 1:1 CBD:THC ratio when spasms are severe. Many patients treating GI discomfort prefer THC-dominant strains with little to no CBD. It's up to your comfort level. If strains that contain high levels of CBD are not effective, switch to strains rich in THC. Sativa strains offer less muscle relaxation than indica strains; therefore, hybrid or indica strains may offer better relief for active spasms.

Cannabigerol (CBG) is the chemical parent to THC and CBD in the raw plant and has been shown to offer substantial benefits for irritable bowel disease (IBD). A recent study out of Italy shows that CBG produced both preventative and curative effects for patients with IBD. That's right. They used a word rarely heard in healthcare—*curative*. CBG reduced the signs of colon injury, decreased inflammatory cytokines, and decreased nitrite production without the negative side effects produced by pharmaceutical agents.[14]

CBG is available in low levels in most strains of cannabis, but breeders are currently developing strains with higher concentrations. Leafly.com lists strains higher in CBG, so patients should be prepared to do some research. Don't be shy about comparing labels at the dispensary to determine which strains offer the highest levels of CBG. Incorporate CBG-rich strains into your daily medicating sessions as much as possible when dealing with GI inflammation and spasms.

Nausea and Vomiting

Nausea, vomiting, and lack of appetite are best treated with THC-rich strains. Be aware that CBD can actually decrease appetite, so if you're dealing with severe nausea and vomiting, you may need to reduce your use of products that contain high amounts of CBD. Strain selection is particularly important when dealing with nausea because the relaxing qualities of hybrid and indica strains are often much more effective at increasing appetite and reducing nausea than many sativa strains.

Patients who do not like the euphoric effect of THC can increase its tolerability by using a 1:1 CBD:THC product or beginning with very low doses of THC and slowly increasing the dosage, as described in Chapter 3, until effective. It can take up to a week for some patients to notice a substantial increase in appetite, so be sure to use adequate doses of THC and be consistent when dosing. One dose of THC every other day may not be adequate to balance the endocannabinoid system, promote healing, and improve appetite. A severe lack of appetite may require moderate doses of THC administered consistently.

For acute nausea and vomiting, the best way to medicate is by inhalation or sublingual administration. It's okay if you need a few more puffs during an episode because higher than normal dosages may be required to overcome active emesis. It is always best to prevent nausea and vomiting than it is to try and overcome it.

Once vomiting is under control, edibles can be dosed around the clock for prevention. As was the case with my patient Andrea, it may take you some time to find the right dose. But once you do, it's a game-changer.

Andrea

Andrea was 28 years old and newly married when she arrived for her consultation with her husband pushing her wheelchair. She described being nauseated 24 hours a day and vomiting up to fifteen times a day, every day. I was shocked. I had never heard of such a thing in an otherwise healthy, young female but soon found out it was called cyclic vomiting syndrome, a diagnosis with no known cause. Andrea barely ate all day and when she did, she typically vomited. At this point, the thought of eating gave her extreme anxiety. She had been to several doctors and tried all the prescription medications available but still suffered every day. At the time, she was on a regimen of ondansetron (Zofran) and prochlorperazine for nausea and vomiting along with tramadol for pain, but the regimen was, obviously, ineffective.

Andrea was not comfortable with inhaling anything since she had never smoked previously, and because her symptoms were around the clock she decided on a sublingual regimen of 5mg of CBD three times a day which was then increased to 10mg three times a day after three days. We started with this protocol because Andrea was initially afraid to take THC, and I thought the CBD might help with bowel inflammation and, therefore, might alleviate her symptoms.

Andrea had no relief after using CBD for seven days, so we decided to add equal amounts of THC to the CBD. She saw immediate changes in her appetite, and the vomiting stopped. She felt so good the first week she began using THC regularly. She actually ate some bacon, which she had been dreaming about for years. (For the record, she said the bacon was a mistake.) After two weeks, she decided to stop using the CBD products altogether because she felt it was not helping her and was an added expense. Andrea increased her dose of THC by 5mg every few days until she felt no nausea and was eating regularly. Once she reached a dose of 40mg of THC taken three times a day, she suffered a seizure. Andrea had no history of seizures, so her current drug therapy was the most likely culprit.

There are reports that THC can act as a pro-convulsant, and possible seizure activity is listed as a side effect of both tramadol and prochlorperazine, the two medications Andrea was taking at the time of her seizure.[15, 16] I contacted her treating physician and informed her that the high dose of THC in addition to the tramadol and prochlorperazine could have contributed to Andrea's seizure. Her doctor agreed and advised Andrea to stop taking the two prescription medications, and I advised Andrea to look for a lower, yet still effective, dosage of THC at the three times a day dosing interval. We had her use indica formulations exclusively, which can offer better relief from nausea. We then monitored her progress.

Andrea tapered off the tramadol and prochlorperazine and was able to decrease her dosage of THC to 20mg every eight hours while still preventing any nausea or vomiting. By removing her ineffective prescription medications and lowering her THC dose, Andrea was a new woman.

When she went to visit her gastroenterologist a couple of months later, he assumed she was using CBD only because she did not appear "high." She told him that she took the same dose of THC three times a day and did not feel intoxicated. It basically became a supplement to keep her endocannabinoid system in balance. It took a bit of time, but cannabis was the one solution that got this young woman's life back on track.

Anal Fissures

Imagine pouring salt and lemon water onto a fresh paper cut. Now imagine the cut is just inside your rectum, and every time you have a bowel movement it's like pouring salt and lemon water onto the wound.

Anal fissures are tears in the delicate lining of the rectum and the result of constipation or frequent diarrhea. Patients suffering from GI disorders frequently suffer from anal fissures too. Treatment involves creams that increase blood flow to the wound, but are often times painfully inadequate (pun intended). Whole-plant cannabis oil has benefits that help reduce pain and promote healing in this delicate area, which makes it an ideal treatment.

Suppositories containing cannabis oil are the best delivery method for treating anal fissures. Unfortunately, cannabis suppositories are not widely available. Patients who are inclined to make their own can do so simply by creating a mixture of cocoa butter and cannabis oil.

You can find suppository molds on Amazon and eBay.

For those who consider making suppositories a bit complicated, there is another, simpler method for patients to compound a diluted cannabis oil to treat and help heal their fissures in the privacy of their home.

- Purchase a syringe of CO_2 extracted, undiluted whole-plant oil with a minimum of 500mg of THC. You can also use 1 gram of a CO_2 extracted concentrate instead. Thin oils are much easier to work with in this recipe than thick or hard oils.
- Pour 1/4 cup of coconut oil into a clean glass jar.
- Melt the coconut oil in the microwave (30 seconds at a time). The oil should be warm but not too hot.
- Place the cannabis oil into the melted coconut oil. Mix until well incorporated. This can take a few minutes, so be patient. Reheat the oil if needed, but *do not* let it get too hot. (Do not go above 240°F.)
- Place the container on the counter to cool.
- If possible, have a bowel movement.
- Take a warm bath with Epsom salts (if tolerated) to help relax the rectum.
- Apply the cannabis-infused oil to the area of the fissure using a finger cot. Be generous with the oil.
- Apply as needed for pain (at least 4 times a day) and after every bowel movement.
- THC administered rectally will be absorbed into the bloodstream but will not cause euphoria. You may feel more relaxed or drowsy, but not high. If concerned, start by using the oil at bedtime.

Cannabis and an upset belly go together like peanut butter and jelly. All along the gastrointestinal tract there are trillions of receptors that work seamlessly with the cannabinoids of the cannabis plant to calm and relax painful symptoms. Cannabis can be used along with current pharmaceutical regimens, or for patients who can't tolerate these drugs, as a first and safe option.

Kaya: the common term
for "marijuana" or
"ganja" in Jamaica.

CHAPTER 18

Glaucoma

*"The current situation and the ongoing disinformation campaign
is dramatically devastative to society not only because the war
on marijuana claims so many victims, but also because it undermines
the trust of millions in their government which is supposed
to act rationally and stay scientifically informed."*

Sebastian Marincolo, PhD[1]
Author and Philosopher

Glaucoma is the second leading cause of irreversible blindness in the world, after age-related disorders. Currently, there are over 3 million people in America, and over 60 million worldwide diagnosed with glaucoma, and more than 120,000 people in the U.S. lose their sight every year.[2] According to the Glaucoma Research Foundation, approximately 10% of people treated for glaucoma will still experience vision loss.[3]

All the way back in 1971, researchers Heplar and Frank found cannabis lowered intraocular pressure, the pressure inside the eye, thereby halting damage to the optic nerve.[4, 5] A healthy eye is bathed in a fluid called aqueous humor, which nourishes the eye while continuously moving in and out of the eye through a series of pathways. This fluid creates the pressure in the eye.

Glaucoma presents when the pressure inside the eye increases above 22mmHG, leading to irreversible damage to the optic nerve. Cannabis decreases intraocular pressure, thereby reducing further damage to the eye and retaining a patient's ability to see.

Pharmaceutical Treatments for Glaucoma

Historically, glaucoma has been treated with a select group of medications that decrease intraocular pressure by decreasing production or increasing outflow of aqueous humor. It seems almost intuitive that medications applied to the eyeball would produce limited systemic side effects, but not so fast. Many patients find it difficult to tolerate available medications and some carry contraindications with cardiac or pulmonary diseases. Surgical interventions for glaucoma have limited success at retention of eyesight.

There has not been a lot of progress regarding glaucoma medications in the last several decades, although two new glaucoma medications, netarsudil (Rhopress) and latanoprostene bunod (Vzulta), were introduced in 2018.[6] Rhopressa is a rho kinase inhibitor that works by enhancing trabecular meshwork outflow, a therapy that was previously abandoned years ago due to adverse side effects. Vzulta contains nitric oxide to dilate blood vessels and is a pro-drug of latanoprost, found in an existing medication called Xalatan, which became available as a generic in 2011.[7] Both of these branded medications will run a patient over $400 a month.

When a drug is about to become available as a generic, look for the appearance of a very similar branded drug (maybe a longer-acting one) to the original. This allows drug companies to maintain brand status (and profits) for their drug. Below, I summarize the most common drugs prescribed for glaucoma.

Beta-blockers are a first-line treatment for many glaucoma patients due to their effectiveness and inexpensive price. Drugs like timolol and levobunolol are widely prescribed and block the activity of epinephrine, which decreases the production of aqueous humor. The most common side effects for this class of drugs are depression and a slowed heart rate. They should be avoided by patients with heart failure, asthma, and insulin dependent diabetes (that's a lot of people).

Epinephrine is used every day in hospitals to treat ventricular fibrillation during a heart attack or for severe allergic reactions. When used for glaucoma, it is administered at much smaller doses to decrease fluid production, resulting in a lower pressure inside the eye. Still, even when used at low doses, epinephrine can cause a rapid heartbeat and is, therefore, prohibited with cardiac patients.

Carbonic anhydrase inhibitors [acetazolamide (Diamox)] come in a capsule and have been around since the 1970s. They are used to decrease production of aqueous humor inside the eye. Unfortunately, these pills have horrible side effects, including nausea, diarrhea, kidney dysfunction, headaches, fatigue, loss of appetite, and blood dyscrasias.

Alpha-2 adrenergic receptor stimulators, or brimonidine, constrict ocular venules and increase oxygen to surrounding tissues. Negative side effects are mild and include inflammation of eye tissues, itching, burning, and eye disturbances, but it is an inexpensive option for treating glaucoma.

Prostaglandin analogs, as mentioned previously, include latanoprost (Xalatan), travoprost (Travatan-Z), and bimatoprost (Lumigan). They increase outflow of aqueous humor and are generally well tolerated. The first drug to market, latanoprost (Xalatan), has been widely prescribed across the globe since 1996 and is currently available in generic form for under $20. Negative side effects include inflamed eyes that are dry, itchy, and sensitive to light. Patients may also experience foreign body sensation, a change in eye color, and pain and stinging with each application. But, when successful, most patients find these drugs very easy to use and affordable.

Pilocarpine is one of the first drugs developed to treat glaucoma but is used more often to dilate the eye during your doctor visits than in ongoing therapy. Pilocarpine stimulates cholinergic receptors and creates a side effect profile difficult for most patients to tolerate. Negative side effects include detachment of the retina, headaches, and vision changes.

Even if patients tolerate these drugs, they may not be effective at lowering intraocular pressure. Latanoprost (generic Xalatan), is one of the most heavily prescribed, and effective, glaucoma medications available today, yet studies show about 25% of patients fail to respond to therapy.[8, 9]

One glaucoma patient who failed conventional therapies was Robert Randall, the first person to prove in court that cannabis was the only medication available which effectively kept him from going blind. Robert discovered problems with his eyesight when he was in college, but his doctor thought he was simply too young to have glaucoma. Robert took the advice offered and went on with his life.

It being the late 1960s, like many college students, Robert regularly used cannabis with friends while pursuing his undergraduate and master's degrees in writing. It was during this time he noticed that when he smoked cannabis his sight improved and the visual disturbances he'd experienced since he was a teen decreased. Of his glaucoma experience, he said: "Since my mid-teens, my evenings had been haunted by minor visual problems-transient tricolored halos. On some evenings I would go white-blind, my vision snared in an impenetrable swirl of absolute illumination-the white void."[10]

Following graduation, Robert moved to Washington State where he was no longer able to find cannabis. His eyesight began to deteriorate quickly. He was referred to Dr. Benjamin Fine, a leading ocular pathologist, who told him his eye pressure was out of control, and he was going blind at the age of 25.

After being treated unsuccessfully with pilocarpine and Diamox, Robert was able to procure a bit of cannabis from a friend. After six months of a self-described "testing period," he realized that when he used cannabis, he experienced none of the telltale signs of increased eye pressure (halos). When he did not use cannabis, the halos reappeared.

Robert's eye pressure stabilized and his progression to blindness came to a halt. With access to cannabis limited and unpredictable, and the cost exceedingly high, he decided to grow a plant in his apartment. He was promptly arrested.

Robert decided to take up the fight to retain his sight in the court system and eventually won a hard-fought battle to become the first legal marijuana smoker in the United States. Robert's medication was supplied to him from a government-owned facility in Mississippi. His case forced the government to acknowledge that it was cannabis, and only cannabis, that was preventing Robert from going blind.

After learning that the government *knew* that marijuana was an effective treatment for the prevention of blindness due to glaucoma, Robert Randall became an outspoken cannabis activist until he died in 2001, never having lost his eyesight.[11]

The Stress of Going Blind

Living with glaucoma can be emotionally, physically, and financially debilitating. The stress of losing one's eyesight, and possible loss of employment, can cause patients to suffer with anxiety and depression.

Craig

The very first patient I saw when the medical dispensaries opened in Connecticut was a glaucoma patient named Craig. He had lost the sight in his left eye and was struggling to keep what remained in his right eye. He was out of medications to try, and the last option his doctor could offer was to have a stint placed into his eye, a solution that would not be completely effective if it worked and was likely to cause partial blindness.

Craig told me that he would smoke about half of a joint in the morning and then press down on his eyes. He said he could actually feel the pressure in his eyes going down. He did not feel the need to re-dose throughout the day. Sometimes at night he would smoke again, but most days he felt the half joint every morning was sufficient. This was confirmed with every doctor visit.

In 1999, researchers found CB1 receptors in the ocular tissues of the human eye, including the ciliary epithelium, the trabecular meshwork, Schlemm's canal, ciliary muscle, ciliary body vessels, and retina. Therefore, endocannabinoid receptors provide an excellent target for new glaucoma therapies.[12] When we consider cannabis as medicine, we need to ask, "How much do I need to use?" Even with the government supplying cannabis to glaucoma patients for 40 years, we still do not have an exact answer.

Determining an effective dosage of cannabinoids for you may require some experimentation. Follow the instructions below and have your doctor measure your intraocular pressure every 1 to 2 weeks until readings are well below 22mmHG.

As we learned by studying medical history, THC is effective at decreasing intraocular pressure. The role of CBD is unknown and may also be effective when combined with THC. (Remember the entourage effect.) Only time and research will provide us with more definitive answers. In the meantime, use strains or products that have at least moderate levels of THC.

Cannabis Treatments for Glaucoma

Cannabis can be administered by any delivery system that is most comfortable: oral, sublingual, or inhaled. Here are some tips for helping to find the right dose of cannabis to decrease intraocular pressure:

1. Begin with a twice a day dosing schedule for inhalation or sublingual delivery methods, 12 hours apart, in order to keep doses lower and blood levels stable. The goal is to always keep sufficient levels of cannabinoids in the bloodstream to prevent further damage to the eye. In studies, THC levels measured after smoking varied from 3 to 27 hours (huge difference!) with higher levels seen when patients used stronger cannabis. I believe dosing every 12 hours is a perfect place to start when treating glaucoma. Increase or decrease the frequency of use based on your measured eye pressure.[13]

2. Write your observations in a journal. Cannabis can affect short-term memory, so you will likely have trouble remembering doses and eye pressures as you experiment before establishing an optimal regimen. Document the amount consumed and frequency of administration. Keep track of your doctor visits in the journal as well.

3. If higher doses of THC are required, or you simply don't tolerate THC at all, consider micro-dosing throughout the day (see Chapter 3). Consuming scheduled, low doses of THC can prevent intoxication while still producing an adequate drop in pressure.

4. If you prefer less pronounced psychoactive side effects, use strains with a high concentration of CBD. Strains with triple or more the amount of CBD to THC will offer less intoxication than THC alone.

5. If you prefer not to inhale, no problem. Oral products produce a longer effect than inhalation, so it may be possible to consume an edible nightly and not have to consume cannabis during the daytime.

Even the government in the District of Columbia superior court had to concede that cannabis is an effective treatment for glaucoma. Strange how it remains unavailable to all patients who need it over 40 years later.

Kush: a subcategory
of the indica strains,
ex: Hindu Kush
or OG Kush.

CHAPTER 19

Sleep, Diabetes, Lyme Disease, and Inflammation of the Prostate

"Health is the first muse, and sleep is the condition to produce it."
Ralph Waldo Emerson[1]
Philosopher and Poet, 1932

Before prohibition took hold at the beginning of the twentieth century, cannabis tincture was readily available in pharmacies as an analgesic, hypnotic, and antispasmodic for the treatment of coughs, sleep disorders, epilepsy, and more.

In this chapter, I summarize some of the emerging science regarding cannabis use as it relates to sleep, diabetes, Lyme disease, and inflammation of the prostate. At first, it may seem as if these conditions have nothing in common. In reality, all but sleep are at least partially the result of chronic, systemic inflammation.

Problems with sleep in this country are rampant and may be a co-condition of another diagnosis or a result of chronic stress. Although limited research exists relating to cannabis use for sleep, cannabis's effectiveness for helping people sleep is legendary. I am always confident when counseling patients that I will be able to help them achieve a restful night's sleep with the use of the right cannabis product.

Although limited research has been done regarding sleep, the endocannabinoid system has been linked to a lack of dreaming, deep relaxation and a reduction in anxiety, often a problem for people dealing with sleep issues.[2] A 2011 study out of California showed patients were able to fall asleep faster when cannabis was used, whether they previously had sleep difficulties or not.[3] Interestingly, I found a study from 1976 which reported a decrease in REM durations after patients were given cannabis extracts, which may be able to explain why cannabis prevents people from dreaming (a positive side effect for PTSD patients that experience nightmares). The problem with this study is in the very high doses used, 70mg to 210mg, which are not typically tolerated by most people.[4] Cannabis gives a dose-related response, and doses like these are just too strong for most people to use comfortably.

Cannabis Treatments for Sleep Disorders

The *International Classification of Sleep Disorders* classifies over 80 different sleep disorders.[5] Nearly 1/3 of the population complains of insomnia, but a much smaller number of people actually have the clinical diagnosis of insomnia. Most people are instead classified with a "sleep disturbance" which includes difficulty falling asleep or waking in the middle of the night.

Sleep disturbances are among the top complaints of patients visiting a cannabis dispensary, often secondary to conditions such as PTSD, pain, cancer, anxiety, and other chronic illness. Many sleep issues can be treated successfully with a relaxing CBD product, while more stubborn sleep disturbances can be quelled by using a terpene-rich, heavily sedating indica strain that's rich in THC. Indica terpenes, such as myrcene, humulene, and linalool, promote deep relaxation.

> **Dr. Richa Love (@drrichalove) May 22**
> One of my patients is 36-yr male veteran who says CBD oil has done wonders for his sleep. He now gets a full night's rest and is less often disturbed by nightmares. Check out this link to learn more about medical cannabis for sleep

Colleen Higgins, R.Ph. (@ColleenHiggy) May 23
That's amazing. Do you know about how many milligrams he needed to take?

Dr. Richa Love (@drrichalove) May 26
Between 60-75mg per day

Colleen Higgins R.Ph. (@ColleenHiggy) May 28 2019 7:02am
Thank you so much![6]

Inhalation for Sleep

Starkiller, Lavender Kush, and God's Gift are deeply relaxing indica strains known to help people fall asleep quickly. Although inhaling cannabis doesn't allow for the same long-acting effects of ingesting an edible, it is often a successful delivery method for people looking to achieve a restful night's sleep. When using an inhaled indica product for sleep, medicate 30 minutes to 1 hour before bedtime. It can take a bit of time for cannabinoids to cause drowsiness and deep relaxation, so using it right at bedtime is not ideal.

If a single medicating session is inadequate, higher blood levels may be necessary. Instead of simply using more at bedtime, smaller doses of a sleepy indica strain used several times throughout the afternoon can be more effective than one large dose delivered right before bedtime, although a larger dose at bedtime may work too. Try medicating every 2–3 hours right up until it's time to go to bed. You are looking to balance the endocannabinoid system to promote deep relaxation. Meditation and deep breathing exercises can help quiet racing thoughts and may help cannabis work better.

For people who wake up every night around 2:00 a.m., a few puffs from your vaporizer along with some meditation can allow the mind to fall back to sleep before becoming fully awake. Keep in mind that if you medicate too close to when your alarm is set to go off, you risk waking up groggy.

How to Use an Edible Product for Sleep

Quality, relaxing CBD oils such, as NuLeaf Naturals, can be effective for mild to moderate sleep problems. Hemp Fusion is a whole-plant CBD capsule for sleep sold on Amazon and has many positive reviews, but this product contains an additional sleep aid called gamma-amino butyric acid (GABA) that contributes to its success. CBD alone may not be powerful enough for people with more stubborn sleep issues. If you have reached doses of 25–75mg CBD per day with no success, it may be time to add or switch to THC.

The effects of cannabis consumed as an edible last longer than when inhaled, so edibles may be ideal for patients who continually wake throughout the night or deal with chronic pain. Indica THC can be combined with CBD when treating anxiety, although whether you want additional CBD for sleep is a matter of personal preference.

To induce sleep, we need to promote deep relaxation of the body and mind through activation and balance of the endocannabinoid system. This can sometimes be a bit tricky. Higher doses of edibles can over-stimulate the endocannabinoid receptor system and have an unintended effect of initially being wakeful (stimulating) rather than sedating. This can leave you staring at the ceiling when you would rather be sleeping.

The ideal way to medicate with a sleep edible is to first medicate with inhaled cannabis in the afternoon (if possible). Medicate with a sleepy indica strain 3–4 hours before bedtime followed by a low-dose edible taken 1 hour before bedtime. Edibles for sleep should be started at 2–5mg and increased every night by 2–5mg until successful. Do not re-medicate with an edible in the middle of the night if not initially successful. Increase your dosage the following night or combine it with other relaxing cannabinoids. Using multiple cannabinoids (THC with CBN) at lower doses may be more effective than a higher dose of a single cannabinoid, in this case, THC.

Patients who require higher doses of THC may be able to reduce their dose if they combine THC with CBN (cannabinol). CBN was initially touted as a heavily relaxing, even sedative, molecule, but the most current research available does not support this conclusion and the relaxing properties attributed to CBN may actually be the result of relaxing terpenes.[7] In my experience, patients who used CBN in our dispensary (it was a relaxing hybrid formula) found it helped them feel less anxious and they achieved a more restful night's sleep. Clearly, further studies are needed.

Combining THC and CBN can help to keep your THC dose lower, which may reduce psychoactive side effects, while still being effective. Kikoko Teas contain chamomile and valerian (both sleep aids) with 3mg of THC and 5mg of CBN to promote a relaxing night's sleep. Always look for products that are indica based and rich in myrcene and linalool.

Cannabis Treatments for Lyme Disease:
A Chronic Inflammatory Condition

Lyme disease is what remains from an infection with a spirochete bacteria, Borrelia burgdorferi, transmitted through a deer tick bite. After treatment with antibiotics, debilitating symptoms can persist for decades, suggesting a prolonged and increased immune response.

The CDC lists chronic symptoms of Lyme disease to be severe headaches, neck stiffness, fatigue, joint pain and swelling, inflammation of the brain and spinal cord, nerve pain, and problems with short-term memory.[8] Once thought to be caused by a neurotoxin released from the bacteria, current research supports the idea that symptoms are caused by a complicated and chronic inflammatory response.

CBD suppresses inflammatory and neuropathic pain and can work as an effective treatment against the symptoms of the disease.[9] It also acts as a neuroprotectant that blocks the formation of nitrotyrosine, a marker that indicates damage to the cells.[10]

THC, also useful to decrease inflammation, can help with symptoms such as nausea, insomnia, anxiety, depression, fatigue, and muscle spasms.

Patients should begin with products low in THC and higher in CBD (10:1 to 5:1 CBD:THC ratio) with a starting CBD dose around 10mg (1–3mg THC), taken 2 to 3 times a day. (See Chapter 3 for how to increase dosages to effective levels.)

If your symptoms require more THC because of severe muscle spasms, nausea, or pain, begin using a product with a 3:1 or 2:1 CBD:THC ratio, although the THC component will feel stronger (10–20mg CBD with 5mg THC). Lyme disease has symptoms that are patient specific. Finding the right product may take a bit of experimentation and time. Don't get discouraged. If you need some extra help, please contact me at SwayInnovations.com so I can help you find the right product in your area.

Cannabis and Diabetes

The American Diabetes Association reports that in 2015 over 30 million Americans had some form of diabetes with associated costs (reported in 2018) above 300 billion dollars.[11] Wow! That is no joke.

Recently, a congressional hearing was held in which insulin drug manufacturers, pharmacy benefit managers, and insurance companies were invited to discuss how the cost of a bottle of insulin has managed to increase from $20 in the year 2000 to over $180 a bottle today.[12] Test strips, which were outrageously priced in 2010 at $100 for one hundred strips are now at almost double that price less than ten years later. It is deplorable, and the best alternative would be to find another approach in order to prevent the development of diabetes.

An overactive endocannabinoid system has been shown to contribute to the development of diabetes and diabetic complications, and is, therefore, a therapeutic target.[13] Rick Simpson, a cannabis advocate who promotes the use of high-dose cannabis oil to treat pain and cancer, reports on his website (phoenixtears.ca) that diabetics who use high-dose cannabis oil find that they may require less insulin during treatment.

Cannabis receptors (CB1 and CB2) have been found in human pancreatic cells, with CB1 receptors found in insulin-producing beta cells, the exact cells that are destroyed in patients with diabetes.[14] Once again, oxidative stress and chronic inflammation play pivotal roles in the development of diabetes and its complications, specifically neuropathy, cardiovascular dysfunction, kidney failure, and damage of the retinas leading to blindness. Excess blood glucose (hyperglycemia) forms reactive oxygen species (ROS) and reactive nitrogen species that directly damage tissues and organs.[15,16] The potent antioxidant CBD may be able to play a role in reducing organ damage during times of high blood glucose.

Cannabinoids contributing the most benefit for diabetes are CBD and THCV, a cannabinoid found to significantly decrease fasting blood glucose as well as improve pancreatic beta-cell function.[17] THC does not appear to have a substantial benefit for diabetes and diabetic complications, possibly because of its well-known ability to increase appetite (aka give users the munchies).

If you begin using CBD and notice an improvement in your blood sugars, I would love to hear from you! Send me a message on Twitter (@ ColleenHiggy) or through my website SwayInnovations.com.

Cannabis and Inflammation of the Prostate

Prostate cancer is the most common cancer in men in the United States. Inflammation of the prostate is often thought to be another sign of aging but is (surprise!) linked to chronic inflammation.

Prostate-specific antigen (PSA) is a protein produced exclusively by prostate cells and may help doctors detect early prostate cancer. A normal PSA is usually less than 4 nanograms per milliliter (ng/mL) of blood.

Although little has been written about cannabinoids lowering the PSA, there are several studies that show the benefits of cannabinoids for inflammation of the prostate and prostate cancer, one of which directly concluded, "cannabinoids should be considered as agents for the management of prostate cancer."[18,19] Expression of CB1 and CB2 receptors was significantly higher in prostate cancer cells and the use of a receptor agonist, such as THC, showed a dose and time-dependent decrease in cell viability.[20]

With these positive findings combined with the high toxicity of current chemotherapy, it is a very real possibility that cannabinoids will be used to treat metastatic prostate cancer in the future.

Considerations When Using Cannabis as Medicine

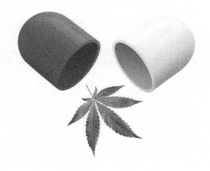

The marijuana industry
has been projected to reach
annual sales of $166 billion
while simultaneously
disrupting industries like
alcohol, tobacco and the
health and wellness industry.

CHAPTER 20

Cost, Withdrawal, and Cannabis Hyperemesis Syndrome

"He's the best physician that knows the worthlessness
of the most medicines."
Ben Franklin[1]
Poor Richard's Almanac 1733

We wrap up our discussion of everything cannabis-related by talking a little about the costs associated with using cannabis as your primary (or secondary) medication, withdrawal effects associated with regular cannabis use, and a syndrome that has presented in emergency rooms more frequently, called Cannabis Hyperemesis Syndrome (CHS). Every drug has positive and negative attributes; cannabis is no exception.

Costs Associated with Cannabis Therapy

With cannabis not legally required to be covered by insurance carriers because of the Schedule 1 federal drug scheduling, the cost of having cannabis in your medical toolbox depends on two factors: your drug tolerance (do you need a little or a lot) and the state in which you reside. When comparing costs around the country, Michigan seemed to have the best prices for cannabis flowers, oils, and edibles. (Go Michigan!) A few puffs a day will have minimal costs, but high, daily doses of professionally manufactured edibles can add up to hundreds of dollars every month. On average, and for most people with a low to moderate tolerance, cannabis will cost between $75 and $300 a month.

For patients who primarily use cannabis flowers to medicate, rolling papers will only run a few dollars. Pipes and bongs can be found for under $50 and, if cleaned regularly, can last for decades.

Patients who are approaching cannabis from a strictly medical perspective typically have no interest in smoking anything. In this case, a quality flower vaporizer will deliver all the benefits of each individual strain without the smoke or smell. A quality flower vaporizer will cost between $100 to $300 and can last for years.

Most dispensaries sell quality cannabis oil cartridges for around $50. If you purchase one cartridge for daytime, another for nighttime, and a $30 Eleaf Istick 20w battery you'll spend $130 total. The average cannabis user will go through one oil vapor cartridge anywhere from seven days (very heavy user) to up to two months (a few puffs per day). Most users find, on average, a cartridge will last around 2 to 4 weeks.

People who exclusively medicate with edibles will save a substantial amount of money if they learn to cook with cannabis. Making your own cannabis butter may seem overwhelming at first, but with machines like the NOVA Decarboxylator ($200 on Amazon) and the Magical Butter Machine ($175 on Amazon), making cannabis butter and tinctures (2-cup minimum) has never been easier. You only need to invest in these machines once, and they will pay for themselves again and again. I recently made an infused coconut butter that contained over 5000mg CBD for only $200. If I was to purchase 5000mg CBD in an oil or tincture at the dispensary, it would easily cost triple that amount.

A top-notch cookbook, such as *The Marijuana Chef Cookbook* by S. T. Oner, is a requirement when learning to make edibles, although YouTube has dozens of instructional videos as well. There is not just one way to make cannabis butter. The most common mistake when cooking edibles is overheating the cannabis thus deactivating the cannabinoids. The motto when cooking with cannabis is to "keep it low and slow." Edibles can be made in bulk and stored in the freezer for 3 to 6 months.

Symptoms of Cannabis Withdrawal

When starting any new medication, it is important to know whether it can be stopped suddenly or should be tapered slowly over the course of one to two weeks. Long-time cannabis users may say that cannabis has zero withdrawal effects, but this is inaccurate. The withdrawal effects can range from mild to very uncomfortable but are not life-threatening.

A 1994 Henningfield study from the National Institute on Drug Abuse (NIDA) showed withdrawal from cannabis to be about equivalent to withdrawal from caffeine.[2] Now, I know some people who love their coffee, but no one is afraid to go to Starbucks because of potential withdrawal. Cannabis produces withdrawal symptoms much milder than those from nicotine, cocaine, or heroin, but a recent study showed some daily users who have a genetic predisposition to addiction can develop a *habit-driven* use that "may strengthen a person's desire to seek the drug."[3]

The severity of withdrawal from cannabis depends on how long and how much you consume on a daily basis. Light cannabis users, a few puffs several times a week, are unlikely to experience significant or noticeable withdrawal effects. Moderate to heavy daily users may experience mild agitation, mild nausea, difficulty sleeping (especially if used for sleep), and headaches. Strenuous exercise, good hydration, yoga, and the herbal supplement Kava Kava can help reduce mild withdrawal symptoms.

Heavy, daily users may experience intense irritability, headaches, night sweats, problems sleeping, a lack of appetite, and nausea (at higher doses). I have spoken with many patients who used cannabis regularly for several years and were able to stop easily, while one heavy concentrate "dabber" described night sweats so severe they needed to change their shirt in the middle of the night. Again, withdrawal symptoms can be unpleasant but will not be life-threatening.

Heavy cannabis users who are concerned about withdrawal symptoms should taper their usage over the course of 1 to 3 weeks. Switching from a full THC product to a 1:1 CBD:THC product can also help people taper their usage more comfortably.

Patients who have been self-medicating with cannabis for an extended period of time may experience an uptick in underlying symptoms such as depression, pain, sleep disturbances, or anxiety. Make a plan for what you will do to compensate for the lost benefits from cannabis. If symptoms become severe, contact your physician to initiate supportive care.

Cannabinoid Hyperemesis Syndrome (CHS)

A 2017 study showed the number of people presenting to emergency rooms with cyclical vomiting and stomach pain has nearly doubled since cannabis was legalized.[4] Even with more people presenting with CHS (which makes sense considering the growing industry), CHS is still considered to be a rare disorder. Cannabinoid Hyperemesis Syndrome has striking similarities to Cyclic Vomiting Syndrome (exactly what it sounds like), so it is possible we may be dealing with a systemic imbalance of cannabinoids.

Some experts question whether the symptoms associated with CHS are the result of nutrients or pesticides used during the growing process. Dr. Michael Verbora, Chief Medical Officer at Aleafia Health in Canada, reported on Twitter that one of his patients switched from an unregulated cannabis product to a regulated product at the same dose and his symptoms resolved.[5]

Cannabinoid Hyperemesis Syndrome is identified scientifically as a condition that develops due to prolonged exposure of cannabinoids that have deactivated the nonselective cation channel TRPV1 of the endocannabinoid receptor. This deactivation leads to severe nausea and vomiting after cannabis is consumed. Patients find relief only from a hot shower or bath, and symptoms resume immediately after re-medicating with cannabis. A recent observational analysis of cannabis-related emergency rooms visits found that more episodes of CHS were attributed to inhalation than to edibles.[6]

A systematic review of CHS by Sorensen et al. identified major diagnostic characteristics in patients with CHS as follows:[7]

- history of regular cannabis use for over a year (74.8%)
- at least weekly cannabis use (97.4%)
- severe nausea and vomiting (100%)
- abdominal pain (85.1%)
- vomiting that recurs in a cyclic pattern over months (100%)
- resolution of symptoms after stopping cannabis (96.8%)
- compulsive hot baths/showers with symptom relief (92.3%)
- male predominance (72.9%)

If a hot shower or bath is the only thing that offers relief from relentless, cyclical stomach pain, nausea, and vomiting, and more cannabis only makes it worse, there is a good chance the diagnosis may be CHS. Those who vomit continuously and can't keep fluids down run the risk of dehydration, so get yourself checked out if symptoms persist.

Mild cases of CHS can be treated by applying an over the counter arthritis cream to the abdomen. Capsaicin cream is made from chili peppers and should be applied in a 4-inch area around the belly button every 4–6 hours until symptoms subside. Because capsaicin is derived from cayenne chilis, it may cause a burning sensation after application. Wash your hands after applying to avoid accidentally touching and burning your eyes.

The only cure for CHS is to stop using cannabis. Cannabis is stored in fat cells and will continue to be slowly released into the bloodstream over time. Heavy users with significant fat stores can find themselves with a positive urine test over a month after they stop using cannabis.

Cannabis Hyperemesis Syndrome is not well understood. If you have switched cannabis producers and are still experiencing CHS symptoms, your body is telling you something. Don't ignore it.

Currently, there are over 30 countries with legal medical cannabis programs including: Argentina, Australia, Canada, Chile, Czech Republic, Denmark, Finland, France, Germany, Greece, Israel, Italy, Mexico, Netherlands, Spain, Switzerland, and Turkey.

Final Thoughts

*"[Cannabis] make you stimulate your mind ... you sit down
and you can meditate and be someone. Rum teach to you
be a drunkard, and herb teach you to be someone."*
Bob Marley[1]

My hope is that this book helps to educate you on the intrinsic medical value of cannabis so you are better able to make an informed decision as to whether cannabis is right for you. The choice to medicate with cannabis, chemotherapy, or any other medical treatment should come only after careful consideration of a therapy's safety, effectiveness, side effects, and cost. Using cannabis as medicine is special in that no Phase 1, 2, or 3 clinical studies exist to determine optimal, precise dosing. Instead, you must *feel* the results. Does pain go away? Does a wound heal? Does anxiety diminish? Are you sleeping better? As a non-toxic drug, safety is not the primary issue. Rather, complete patient satisfaction is the measure of success. Refreshing, when you think about it.

Throughout the chapters in this book, I have guided you about how to safely and comfortably begin using THC, CBD, CBN and THCA in order to treat different issues, but not once did I provide a single dose to which you must adhere. I recommended comfortable starting doses and intervals when to take more if desired.

Cannabis can be increased and decreased as needed. In this way, it's like insulin. If a person with diabetes ate the exact same foods every day and took the exact same dose of insulin, they could still have blood glucose numbers that fluctuate for no rhyme or reason. This is because the body is constantly in flux, and the way to use cannabis properly is to listen to your body in order to establish a state of homeostasis through a combination of food, exercise, mindset, love, and medicine, for starters. Well-designed drug studies can help to establish treatment parameters for chronic, systemic inflammation, but for now, your satisfaction is the measurement of success.

How does someone know they are balanced? Easy, they feel good. They feel relaxed. Anything else is not balanced.

Somehow, and with direct intent, the pharmaceutical industry has become the singular, dominant voice regarding how we treat disease in the United States. When you visit your doctor, you almost expect to leave with at least one prescription or consider it a waste of time. How did this happen? How did the United States become the most medicated country in the world, yet is listed as number 43 for life expectancy? Billions in advertising dollars will have you believe that better living through chemistry is possible, but the reality is that every drug has its price whether it be in dollars or deadly side effects.

For those who put their trust in our government-regulated healthcare system the decision about whether to try cannabis, or any alternative therapy for that matter, can be a confusing one. When the former Attorney General of the United States, Jeff Sessions, is quoted as saying "Good people don't smoke marijuana," that cuts deep.[2] It is a gross misstatement by an ignorant government official that keeps the propaganda of Harry Anslinger alive 80 years after it was first put forward.

Let's not forget, the legalization of cannabis did not get where it is today with the help of the government but despite it. The citizens of California, Colorado, and Washington were no longer willing to accept cannabis prohibition and started a wave of legalization that spread across the country like wildfire. People have been waiting for the return of legal cannabis, and in less than a decade the cannabis industry has morphed into a worldwide, multibillion-dollar industry that continues to expand every year.

Besides helping with a multitude of symptoms, cannabis targets disease from a different vantage point, one where altering the endocan-nabinoid receptor system can affect underlying development of diseases like Alzheimer's disease, Parkinson's disease and multiple sclerosis—all for pennies on the pharmaceutical dollar.

The approach of treating the root cause of disease has arrived for the pharmaceutical industry with the approval of Zolgensma, a new gene therapy drug for a rare childhood disorder called spinal muscular at-rophy. The FDA approved Zolgensma in 2019, and it has been called a "miracle drug." But miracles don't come cheap in the United States. It will cost patients up to 2.1 million dollars a year.[3] This kind of pricing struc-ture affects every single citizen of this country. So, while it is possible in some cases to treat the root cause of disease through pharmacology, it will cost you big time!

The winds of change are shifting the public perspective. Healing with medicinal plants is as old as mankind itself and has been documented extensively. Cannabis is, first and foremost, safe. As David Schmader, author of *Weed: The User's Guide*, writes, "Even aspirin can kill you if you take too much, but a fatal dose of marijuana would require ingestion of fifteen hundred pounds in fifteen minutes—a physical impossibility for any human, even Snoop Dogg."[4]

If you're staring at a pile of pill bottles and wondering, "How did I get here?" it may be time to try the natural, yet powerful relief offered by cannabis. It is safe. It has been used by humans for millennia. And you can trust the One who made it.

Acknowledgments

This book was just an idea in my head and would not exist without the support, love, and amazing skills of the following people:

Grace, for suffering through another night of pizza so I could squeeze out "just one more thing;"

Julie and Andrea for your unwavering support and belief in my abilities to fly;

Craig for being my hero by helping to get this book across the finish line (amazing job)

Michael, for never being shocked by what I try and accomplish on a whim;

Cristen Iris for your work as my developmental editor—I handed you a mess, and you created structure and an actual, readable book;

David Provolo for creating the beautiful cover and interior design;

My sister Aimee for her love, encouragement and support along with a great cover photo;

Most importantly, the patients who allow me to help guide and assist them on their medical journey—your ability to keep moving forward in the face of adversity keeps me motivated to do what I do!

Notes

Introduction

1 Hippocrates Quotes. BrainyQuote.com, BrainyMedia Inc, 2019. https://www.brainyquote.com/quotes/hippocrates_133221, accessed September 30, 2019.

2 A Look at Drug Spending in the U.S. Estimates and projections from various stakeholders. Pewtrusts.org. The Pew Charitable Trusts, 2019. https://www.pewtrusts.org/it/research-and-analysis/fact-sheets/2018/02/a-look-at-drug-spending-in-the-uson 8/29/18, accessed October 3, 2019.

3 Nearly 7 in 10 Americans Take Prescription Drugs. Mayo Clinic, Olmsted Medical Center Find. NewsNetwork.MayoClinic.org, Mayo Clinic, 2019. https://news-network.mayoclinic.org/discussion/nearly-7-in-10-americans-take-prescription-drugs-mayo-clinic-olmsted-medical-center-find/, accessed October 3, 2019.

4 The World Fact book, Country Comparison: Life Expectancy at Birth. CIA.gov, Central Intelligence Agency, 2019. 9/1/2019. https://www.cia.gov/about-cia/site-policies/#copy, accessed October 3, 2019.

Chapter 1

1 Jefferson, Thomas in Eternal Foe of Murray. *The Joy of Words.* J.G. Ferguson Publishing Co. 1960, pg 122.

2 420 Day: Why There Are So Many Different Names for Weed by Katy Steinmetz. time.com, Time USA, LLC, 2019. https://time.com/4747501/420-day-weed-marijuana-pot-slang/April 20, 2017, accessed October 3, 2019.

3 George Washington Letter To William Pearce - August 17, 1794. MountVernon.org, Mount Vernon Ladies' Association, 2019. https://www.mountvernon.org/education/primary-sources-2/article/george-washington-letter-to-william-pearce--august-17-1794/, accessed October 3, 2019.

4 Hemp & Flax in Colonial America by Ben Swenson. history.org, The Colonial Williamsburg Foundation, 2019. https://www.history.org/foundation/journal/winter15/hemp.cfm, accessed October 3, 2019.

5 "Ford Shows Auto Built of Plastic - Strong Material Derived from Soy Beans, Wheat, Corn is used for Body and Fenders," *New York Times*, 14 August 1941.

6 Reefer Madness by Andy Fickman, howlingpixel.com, Howling Pixel, 2019. https://howlingpixel.com/i-en/Reefer_Madness#cite_note-History-5, accessed October 23, 2019.

7 Mayor's Committee on Marijuana, by the New York Academy of Medicine, "The Laguardia Committee Report", druglibrary.com, Drug Library, 2019. http://www.druglibrary.org/schaffer/library/studies/lag/lagmenu.htm, accessed October 21, 2019.

8 The man behind the marijuana ban for all the wrong reasons by Cydney Adams. CBSNews.com, CBS Interactive Inc., 2019. https://www.cbsnews.com/news/harry-anslinger-the-man-behind-the-marijuana-ban/, accessed October 3, 2019.

9 Leary v. United States, 395 U.S. 6 (1969), supreme.justia.com, Justia, 2019. https://supreme.justia.com/cases/federal/us/395/6/, accessed October 21, 2019.

10 Understanding Drug Schedules. HealthyChildren.Org, American Academy of Pediatrics, 2019. https://www.healthychildren.org/English/ages-stages/teen/substance-abuse/Pages/Controlled-Substances-Not-Just-Street-Drugs.aspx, accessed October 3, 2019.

11 Marijuana: A Signal of Misunderstanding. *The Official Report of the National Commission on Marihuana and Drug Abuse*, by The New American Library, INC. 1972.

12 Federal IND Patients: Recipients of Legal Medical Cannabis, provided by the U.S. government under the Investigational New Drug Program (Compassionate Access I.N.D.), medicalcannabis.com, Patients Out of Time, 2018. https://www.medicalcannabis.com/patients-care-givers/federal-ind-patients/, accessed October 24, 2019.

13 About six in ten Americans support legalization by Hannah Hartig and Abigail Geiger. PewResearch.com, Pew Research Center, 2019. https://www.pewresearch.org/fact-tank/2018/10/08/americans-support-marijuana-legalization/, accessed October 3, 2019.

14 Alcohol Sales Dropped 15% In States With Medical Marijuana Laws by Thomas Pellechia. forbes.com. Forbes Inc, 2019. https://www.forbes.com/sites/jeffarnold/2019/10/03/joe-girardi-david-ross-hope-to-catch-on-as-cubs-managerial-contenders/#738a56803068, accessed October 3, 2019.

15 Current health expenditure (% of GDP). data.worldbank.org, The World Bank, 2019. https://data.worldbank.org/indicator/SH.XPD.CHEX.GD.ZS, accessed October 3, 2019.

16 The World Fact book. Country Comparison: Life Expectancy at Birth. CIA.gov, Central Intelligence Agency, 2019. 9/1/2019. https://www.cia.gov/about-cia/site-policies/#copy, accessed October 3, 2019.

17 Did the FDA Ignite the Opioid Epidemic? Bill Whitaker reporting for CBS News, cbsnews.com, CBS Interactive Inc., 2019. https://www.cbsnews.com/video/opioid-epidemic-did-the-fda-ignite-the-crisis-60-minutes/, accessed October 3, 2019.

18 Promoting Safe and Effective Drugs for 100 Years by Michelle Meadows. FDA. gov, U.S. Food and Drug Administration, https://www.fda.gov/media/109488/download, accessed October 3, 2019.

19 Did the FDA Ignite the Opioid Epidemic? with Bill Whitaker. CBSnews.com, CBS Interactive Inc., 2019. https://www.cbsnews.com/news/opioid-epidemic-did-the-fda-ignite-the-crisis-60-minutes/, accessed October 3, 2019.

20 Macy, Beth. *Dopesick Dealers, Doctors, and the Drug Company that Addicted America*, Little Brown and Company, 2018 pp 63-64.

21 Did the FDA Ignite the Opioid Epidemic? with Bill Whitaker. CBSnews.com, CBS Interactive Inc., 2019. https://www.cbsnews.com/news/opioid-epidemic-did-the-fda-ignite-the-crisis-60-minutes/, accessed October 3, 2019.

22 GW Pharmaceuticals Press Release, ir.gwpharma.com, GW Pharmcaeuticals plc, 2019. http://ir.gwpharm.com/news-releases/news-release-details/epidiolexr-cannabidiol-oral-solution-first-fda-approved-plant, accessed October 3, 2019.

23 Schedules of Controlled Substances: Placement in Schedule V of Certain FDA-Approved Drugs Containing Cannabidiol; Corresponding Change to Permit Requirements, federalregister.gov, Drug Enforcement Administration, 2019. https://www.federalregister.gov/documents/2018/09/28/2018-21121/schedules-of-controlled-substances-placement-in-schedule-v-of-certain-fda-approved-drugs-containing, accessed October 3, 2019.

24 Industrial Hemp, nifa.usda.gov, United States Department of Agriculture, 2019. https://nifa.usda.gov/industrial-hemp, accessed October 21, 2019.

25 Valsartan Recall: FDA Issues Warning to API Manufacturer. PharmacyTimes. com, Pharmacy & Healthcare Communications, LLC,, 2019.https://www.pharmacytimes.com/resource-centers/cardiovascular-health/valsartan-recall-fda-issues-warning-to-api-manufacturer, accessed October 3, 2019.

Chapter 2

1 US Dept of Justice, DEA. Marijuana Rescheduling Petition, Docket No. 86-22 Opinion and Recommended Ruling, Findings of Fact, Conclusions of Law and Decision of Administrative Law Judge Francis L. Young, Administrative Law Judge Dated: September 6, 1988 druglibrary.org, Schaffer Library of Drug Policy, 2019. http://www.druglibrary.org/schaffer/Library/studies/YOUNG/index.html, accessed October 3, 2019.

2 Komorowski J., Stepień H. "The role of the endocannabinoid system in the regulation of endocrine function and in the control of energy balance in humans." *Postepy Hig Med Dosw* (Online). 2007; 61:99-105.

3 Kerstin Iffland, Michael Carus and Dr. Franjo Grotenhermen. "Decarboxylation of Tetrahydrocannabinolic acid (THCA) to active THC." *European Industrial Hemp Association* (EIHA) 2019.

4 E M Rock, R L Kopstick, C L Limebeer, and L A Parker. "Tetrahydrocannabinolic acid reduces nausea-induced conditioned gaping in rats and vomiting in Suncus murinus." *British Journal Pharmacology.* 2013 Oct;170(3): 641–648.

5 Peter M. Zygmunt, David A. Andersson and Edward D. Högestätt. "Δ9-Tetrahydrocannabinol and Cannabinol Activate Capsaicin-Sensitive Sensory Nerves via a CB1 and CB2 Cannabinoid Receptor-Independent Mechanism." *Journal of Neuroscience* 1 June 2002, 22 (11) 4720-4727.

6 DEA Rules 1999, Drug Enforcement Administration, 2019. https://www.deadiversion.usdoj.gov/fed_regs/rules/1999/fr0702.htm, accessed October 3, 2019.

7 Ethan B. Russo. "Taming THC: potential cannabis synergy and phytocannabinoid-terpenoid entourage effects." *Br J Pharmacol.* 2011 Aug; 163(7):1344–1364.

Chapter 3

1 Dr. Sanjay Gupta to Jeff Sessions: Medical marijuana could save many addicted to opioids, CNN.com, Cable News Network, 2019. https://www.cnn.com/2018/04/24/health/medical-marijuana-opioid-epidemic-sanjay-gupta/index.html, accessed October 3, 2019.

2 Maroon, Joseph and Bost, Jeff. "Review of the neurological benefits of phytocannabinoids" *Surg Neurol Int.* 2018; 9: 91.

3 Yamaori S, Okamoto Y, Yamamoto I, Watanabe K. "Cannabidiol, a major phytocannabinoid, as a potent atypical inhibitor for CYP2D6." *Drug Metab Dispos.* 2011;39:2049–56.

4 Jiang R, Yamaori S, Okamoto Y, Yamamoto I, Watanabe K. "Cannabidiol is a potent inhibitor of the catalytic activity of cytochrome P450 2C19." *Drug Metab Pharmacokinet.* 2013; 28:332–8.

5 Zendulka O, Dovrtělová G, Nosková K, et al. "Cannabinoids and cytochrome P450 interactions." *Curr Drug Metab.* 2016;17:206–26.

6 Arellano AL, Papaseit E, Romaguera A, Torrens M, Farré M. "Neuropsychiatric and general interactions of natural and synthetic cannabinoids with drugs of abuse and medicines." *CNS Neurol Disord Drug Targets.* 2017;16(5):554-566.

7 Gaston TE, Bebin EM, Cutter GR, Liu Y, Szaflarski JP. "UAB CBD Program. Interactions between cannabidiol and commonly used anti- epileptic drugs." *Epilepsia* 2017;581586-92.

8 Geffrey AL, Pollack SF, Bruno PL, Thiele EA. "Drug-drug interaction be- tween clobazam and cannabidiol in children with refractory epilepsy." *Epilepsia* 2015;56:1246-51.

9 Stott C, White L, Wright S, Wilbraham D, Guy G. "A phase I, open-la- bel, randomized, crossover study in three parallel groups to evaluate the effect of rifampicin, ketoconazole, and omeprazole on the phar-macokinetics of THC/CBD oromucosal spray in healthy volunteers." *Springerplus* 2013;2:236.

10 Jane Carlisle Maxwell, PhD and Bruce Mendelson, MPA, "What do we know about the impact of the laws related to marijuana?" *J Addict Med.* 2016 Feb; 10(1):3-12.

11 Marinol: Highlights of Prescribing Information. accessdata.fda.gov, US Food and Drug Administration, 2019. https://www.accessdata.fda.gov/drugsatfda_docs/label/2017/018651s029lbl.pdf, accessed October 3, 2019.

12 Rainer Hambrecht, MD, FESC; Kathy Berra, MSN, ANP; Karen J. Calfas, PhD, "Managing Your Angina Symptoms With Nitroglycerin What About Exercise?" ahajournals.org, *Circulation, Cardiology Patient* Page e642-645.

13 Millar, Sophie A., Stone, Nicole L., Yates, Andrew S., and O'Sullivan, Saoirse E. "A Systematic Review on the Pharmacokinetics of Cannabidiol in Humans." *Front Pharmacol.* 2018; 9: 1365.

14 Huestis, Marikyn. "Human Cannabinoid Pharmacokinetics." *Chem Biodivers* 2007 Aug, 4(8):1770-1804.

Chapter 4

1 David L. Bearman, MD Biography phone interview Mar. 1, 2006. MedicalMarijuan.procon.org, procon.org, 2019. https://medicalmarijuana.procon.org/view.source.php?sourceID=000594, accessed October 3, 2019.

2 Tashkin, Donald P. "Effects of Marijuana Smoking on the Lung." *Annals of the American Thoracic Society,* Vol. 10, No. 3, June 1, 2013.

3 Mark J. Pletcher, MD, MPH; Eric Vittinghoff, PhD; Ravi Kalhan, MD, MS, Joshua Richman, MD, PhD; Monika Safford, MD; Stephen Sidney, MD, MPH; Feng Lin, MS; Stefan Kertesz, MD. "Association Between Marijuana Exposure and Pulmonary Function Over 20 Years." *JAMA.* 2012;307(2):173-181.

4 Pure Pressure Half Lb of herb into 60 grams of Rosin, Youtube.com, Google LLC, 2019. https://www.youtube.com/watch?v=AebhmH5k1SA&t=155s, accessed October 2019.

5 How to Take a Dab (Dabbing Tutorial), m, Google LLC, 2019. https://www.youtube.com/watch?v=UrlW8dcSWcs, accessed October 3, 2019.

6 25 Best Inventions of 2016. time.com, Time USA LLC, 2019. https://time.com/4572079/best-inventions-2016/, accessed October 3, 2019.

Chapter 5

1 Marincolo, Sebastian. *high: insights on marijuana*, Dog Ear Press 2010, pg 203.

Chapter 6

1 Reed, Lawrence. *Real Heroes: Inspiring True Stories of Courage, Character, and Conviction*, ISI Books. Sept 27, 2016, pp 241-243.

2 Andrew A. Monte, MD, PhD; Shelby K. Shelton, MPH; Eleanor Mills, BS; Jessica Saben, PhD; Andrew Hopkinson, BS; Brandon Sonn, MS; Michael Devivo, BA; Tae Chang, MD; Jacob Fox, BA; Cody Brevik, MD; Kayla Williamson, MS; and Diana Abbott, PhD. "Acute Illness Associated With Cannabis Use, by Route of Exposure. An Observational Study." *Annals of Internal Medicine* 2019;170:531-537.

3 Huestis, Marilyn. "Human Cannabinoid Pharmacokinetics." *Chem Biodivers.* 2007 Aug; 4(8): 1770–1804.

4 Andrew A. Monte, MD, PhD; Shelby K. Shelton, MPH; Eleanor Mills, BS; Jessica Saben, PhD; Andrew Hopkinson, BS; Brandon Sonn, MS; Michael Devivo, BA; Tae Chang, MD; Jacob Fox, BA; Cody Brevik, MD; Kayla Williamson, MS; Diana Abbott, PhD. "Acute Illness Associated With Cannabis Use, by Route of Exposure: An Observational Study." *Annals of Internal Medicine*;16 April 2019.

5 Hartman, Rececca L, Brown, Timothy L, Milavetz, Gary, Spurgin, Andrew, Gorelick, David A, Gaffney, Gary, Huestis, Marilyn A. "Controlled Cannabis Vaporizer Administration: Blood and Plasma Cannabinoids with and without Alcohol" *Clinical Chemistry*: May 2015.

Chapter 7

1 Grinspoon MD, Lester, Bakalar, James B. *Marihuana The Forbidden Medicine,* Yale University Press, 1997, pg. 283.

2 Ständer S1, Schmelz M, Metze D, Luger T, Rukwied R. "Distribution of cannabinoid receptor 1 (CB1) and 2 (CB2) on sensory nerve fibers and adnexal structures in human skin." *J Dermatol Sci.* 2005 Jun;38(3):177-88.

3 Chelliah MP, Zinn Z, Khuu P, Teng JMC. "Self-initiated use of topical cannabidiol oil for epidermolysis bullosa." *Pediatr Dermatol.* 2018 Jul;35(4):e224-e227.

4 Jessica S. Mounessa, BSa,b, Julia A. Siegel, BAc, Cory A. Dunnick, MDa,b, Robert P. Dellavalle, MD, PhD, MSPHa. "The role of cannabinoids in dermatology." *J Am Acad Dermatol.* July 2017 Volume 77, Issue 1, Pages 188–190.

5 A Frankova, A Janatova, J Tauchen, L Kokoska. "In vitro Antimicrobial and Antioxidant Activity of Extracts from Six Chemotypes of Medicinal Cannabis." *Planta Med* 2016; 82(S 01): S1-S38.

6 Bacterial Skin Infections: Impetigo and MRSA. health.Ny.gov, New York State Department of Health, https://www.health.ny.gov/diseases/communicable/athletic_skin_infections/bacterial.htm, accessed October 3, 2019.

7 Chakraborty S1, Afaq N1, Singh N1, Majumdar S. "Antimicrobial activity of Cannabis sativa, Thuja orientalis and Psidium guajava leaf extracts against methicillin-resistant Staphylococcus aureus." *J Integr Med.* 2018 Sep;16(5):350-357.

8 Group A Streptococcal (GAS) Disease. Necrotizing Fasciitis: All you need to know. CDC.gov, US Department of Health & Human Services, 2019. https://www.cdc.gov/groupastrep/diseases-public/necrotizing-fasciitis.html. accessed October 3, 2019.

9 Focht DR 3rd, Spicer C, Fairchok MP. "The efficacy of duct tape vs cryotherapy in the treatment of verruca vulgaris (the common wart)." *Arch Pediatric Adolesc Med.*, 2002 Oct; 156(10):971-4.

10 Appendino G1, Gibbons S, Giana A, Pagani A, Grassi G, Stavri M, Smith E, Rahman MM. "Antibacterial cannabinoids from Cannabis sativa: a structure-activity study." *J Nat Prod.* 2008 Aug;71(8):1427-30.

Chapter 8

1 Use of Cannabis Medicines in Clinical Practice by David Hadorn MD PhD. medicalmarijuana.procon.org, PDF, https://medicalmarijuana.procon.org/sourcefiles/use-of-cannabis-medicines-in-clinical-practice.pdf, accessed October 3, 2019.

2 James Dahlhamer, PhD, Jacqueline Lucas, MPH, Carla Zelaya, PhD, Richard Nahin, PhD, Sean Mackey, MD, Ph D, Lynn DeBar, PhD, Robert Kerns, PhD, Michael Von Korff, ScD, Linda Porter, PhD, Charles Helmick, MD. "Prevalence of Chronic Pain and High-Impact Chronic Pain Among Adults — United States, 2016." *CDC Morbidity and Mortality Weekly Report*, September 14, 2018 / 67(36);1001–1006.

3 Johns Hopkins Medicine Blaustein Pain Treatment Center. "Types of Pain We Treat." HopkinsMedicine.org, The Johns Hopkins University, The Johns Hopkins Hospital, and Johns Hopkins Health System, 2019. https://www.hopkinsmedicine.org/pain/blaustein_pain_center/index.html, accessed October 3, 2019.

4 Merck Manual Consumer Version, Nociceptive Pain by James C Watson, MD, Mayo Clinic, merckmanuals.com, Merck Sharp & Dohme Corp. 2019. https://www.merckmanuals.com/home/brain,-spinal-cord,-and-nerve-disorders/pain/nociceptive-pain, accessed October 21, 2019.

5 Andrew Rosenblum, Lisa A. Marsch, Herman Joseph, and Russell K. Portenoy. "Opioids and the Treatment of Chronic Pain: Controversies, Current Status, and Future Directions." *Experimental and Clinical Psychopharmacology*, 2008 Oct; 16(5): 405–416.

6 Thomas R. Kosten, M.D.1,2 and Tony P. George, M.D.1,3, "The Neurobiology of Opioid Dependence: Implications for Treatment." *Sci Pract Perspect.* 2002 Jul; 1(1): 13–20.

7 Feng Y, He X, Yang Y, Chao D, Lazarus LH, Xia Y. "Current research on Opioid Receptor Function." *Curr Drug Targets* 2012 Feb;13(2):230-46.

8 Dr. Jack E. Henningfield of the National Institute of Drug Abuse (NIDA) and Dr. Neal L. Benowitz of the University of California at San Francisco (UCSF), data from an article in the New York Times (August 2, 1994, p. C3).

9 Provisional Drug Overdose Death Counts. CDC.gov, Centers for Disease Control and Prevention, 2019. https://www.cdc.gov/nchs/nvss/vsrr/drug-overdose-data.htm, accessed October 3, 2019.

10 Shenglong Zou and Ujendra Kumar. "Cannabinoid Receptors and the Endocannabinoid System: Signaling and Function in the Central Nervous System." *Int J Mol Sci.* 2018 Mar; 19(3): 833.

11 Sascha Dublin, MD, PhD,a,b Rod L. Walker, MS,a Shelly L. Gray, PharmD, MS,c Rebecca A. Hubbard, PhD,e Melissa L. Anderson, MS,a Onchee Yu, MS,a Paul K. Crane, MD, MPH,d and Eric B. Larson, MD, MPHa,d. "Prescription Opioids and Risk of Dementia or Cognitive Decline: A Prospective Cohort Study." *J Am Geriatr Soc.* 2015 Aug; 63(8): 1519–1526.

12 Kevin F. Boehnke, J. Ryan Scott, Evangelos Litinas, Suzanne Sisley, David A. Williams, Daniel J. Clauw. "Pills to pot: observational analyses of cannabis substitution among medical cannabis users with chronic pain." *The Journal of Pain* 2019 Jul;20(7);830-841.

13 A Guide to Drug Safety Terms at FDA. FDA.gov, Food and Drug Administration, 2019. https://www.fda.gov/media/74382/download, accessed October 3, 2019.

14 Russell IJ1, Orr MD, Littman B, Vipraio GA, Alboukrek D, Michalek JE, Lopez Y, MacKillip F. "Elevated cerebrospinal fluid levels of substance P in patients with the fibromyalgia syndrome." *Arthritis Rheum.* 1994 Nov;37(11):1593-601.

15 Karen Bandeen-Roche,1 Jeremy D. Walston,2 Yi Huang,3 Richard D. Semba,4 and Luigi Ferrucci5. "Measuring Systemic Inflammatory Regulation in Older Adults: Evidence and Utility." *Rejuvenation Res.* 2009 Dec; 12(6): 403–410.

16 Stephen D. Anton,1 Keelin Moehl,2 William T. Donahoo,3 Krisztina Marosi,2 Stephanie Lee,1 Arch G. Mainous, III,4 Christiaan Leeuwenburgh,1 and Mark P. Mattson2,5. "Flipping the Metabolic Switch: Understanding and Applying Health Benefits of Fasting." *Obesity* (Silver Spring). 2018 Feb; 26(2): 254–268.

17 Sumner Burstein. "Cannabidiol (CBD) and its analogs: a review of their effects on inflammation." *Bioorganic and Medicinal Chemistry* 23 (2015) 1377-1385.

18 Russell IJ, Vipraio G, Fletcher EM, Lopez YM, Orr MD, Michalek JE. "Characteristics of spinal fluid (CSF) substance p (SP) and calcitonin gene related peptide (CGRP) in fibromyalgia syndrome." (FMS) *Arthritis & Rheumatism*. 1996;39:S275.

19 Russell IJ. "Neurochemical pathogenesis of fibromyalgia." *Zeitschrift fur Rheumatologie*. 1998;57(Suppl 2):63–66.

20 Schwarz MJ, Spath M, Muller-Bardorff H, Pongratz DE, Bondy B, Ackenheil M. "Relationship of substance P, 5-hydroxyindole acetic acid and tryptophan in serum of fibromyalgia patients." *Neuroscience Letters*. 1999;259:196–198.

21 Inanici F, Yunus MB. "History of fibromyalgia:past to present." *Curr Pain Headache Rep*. 2004 Oct;8(5):369-78.

22 Fibromyalgia by Tara E. Dymon Pharm D. *Neurologic and Psychiatric Care I*, ACSAP-PDF, (accp.com), 2019. https://www.accp.com/docs/bookstore/acsap/a15b1_m1sample.pdf, accessed October 3, 2019.

23 Fibromyalgia. MayoClinic.org, Mayo Foundation for Medical Education and Research (MFMER), 2019. https://www.mayoclinic.org/diseases-conditions/fibromyalgia/diagnosis-treatment/drc-20354785, accessed October 3, 2019.

Chapter 9

1 Hecht, Peter. "Former Surgeon General calls for marijuana acceptance." *The Sacramento Bee,* Feb 13, 2016.

2 Evolution of Cancer Treatments: Chemotherapy. cancer.org, American Cancer Society, Inc. 2019, https://www.cancer.org/cancer/cancer-basics/history-of-cancer/cancer-treatment-chemo.html, accessed October 3, 2019.

3 Martin R Tramèr, Dawn Carroll, Fiona A Campbell, D John M Reynolds, R Andrew Moore, Henry J McQuay. "Cannabinoids for control of chemotherapy induced nausea and vomiting: quantitative systematic review." *BMJ* Volume 323 (7) July 2001.

4 EM Rock,1 D Bolognini,2 CL Limebeer,1 MG Cascio,2 S Anavi-Goffer,2 PJ Fletcher,3 R Mechoulam,4 RG Pertwee,2 and LA Parker1. "Cannabidiol, a non-psychotropic component of cannabis, attenuates vomiting and nausea-like behaviour via indirect agonism of 5-HT1A somatodendritic autoreceptors in the dorsal raphe nucleus." *British Journal Pharmacology*. 2012 Apr; 165(8): 2620-2634.

5 Ethan B Russo. "Cannabinoids in the management of difficult to treat pain." *Ther Clin Risk Manag*. 2008 Feb; 4(1): 245-259.

6 Ward SJ1, McAllister SD, Kawamura R, Murase R, Neelakantan H, Walker EA. "Cannabidiol inhibits paclitaxel-induced neuropathic pain through 5-HT(1A) receptors without diminishing nervous system function or chemotherapy efficacy." *Br J Pharmacol*. 2014 Feb;171(3):636-45.

7 Zhao ZB, Guan DW, Liu WW, Wang T, Fan YY, Cheng ZH, Zheng JL, Hu GY Fa yi xue za zhi. "Expression of cannabinoid receptor I during mice skin incised wound healing course." *Chemo-EuropePMC*. [01 Aug 2010, 26(4):241-245].

8 Terézia Kisková, Felicitas Mungenast, Mária Suváková, Walter Jäger, and Theresia Thalhammer. "Future Aspects for Cannabinoids in Breast Cancer Therapy." *Int J Mol Sc*i. 2019 Apr; 20(7): 1673.

9 Giovanni Appendino, Simon Gibbons, Anna Giana, Alberto Pagani, Gianpaolo Grassi, Michael Stavri, Eileen Smith, M. Mukhlesur Rahman. "Antibacterial Cannabinoids from Cannabis sativa: A Structure–Activity Study." *J. Nat.Prod*. 2008, 71,8,1427-1430.

10 Surang Leelawat, Kawin Leelawat, Siriluck Narong, and Orphan Matangkasombut. "The Dual Effects of Delta-9- tetrahydrocannabidiol on Cholangiocarcinoma Cells: Anti-Invasion Activity at Low Concentration and Apoptosis Induction at High Concentration." *Cancer Investigation*, May 2010, 120(5):357-63.

11 Liu WM, Scott KA, Shamash J, Joel S and Powles TB. "Enhancing the *in vitro* cytotoxic activity of delta-9-tetrahydrocnnabidiol in leukemia cells through a combinatorial approach." *Leuk Lymphoma* 49: 1800-1809, 2008.

12 Shrivastava A, Kuzontkoski PM, Groopman JE and Prasad A. "Cannabidiol indices programmed cell death in breast cancer cells by coordinating the cross-talk between apoptosis and autphagy." *Mol Cancer Ther* 10: 1161-1172, 2011.

13 Massi P, Solinas M, Cinquina V and Parolaro D. "Cannabidiol as potential anti-cancer drug." *British Journal of Clinical Pharmacology* 75; 303-312, 2013.

14 John M McPartland, Marnis Duncan, Vincenzo Di Marzo, and Roger G Pertwee. "Are cannabidiol and Δ 9-tetrahydrocannabivarin negative modulators of the endocannabinoid system? A systemic review." *British Journal of Pharmacology*, 2015 Feb, 172(3):737-753.

15 Katherine Ann Scott, Sini Shah, Angus George Dalgleish and Wai Man Liu. "Enhancing the Activity of Cannabidiol and other Cannabinoids In Vitro Through Modifications to Drug Combinations and Treatment Schedules." *Anticancer Research* 33: 4373-4380 (2013).

16 George W. Booz, "Cannabidiol as an Emergent Therapeutic Strategy for Lessening the Impact of Inflammation on Oxidative Stress." *Free Radic Biol Med.* 2011 Sep 1; 51(5): 1054–1061.

17 Hao Pan, Partha Mukhopadhyay, Mohanraj Rajesh, Vivek Patel, Bani Mukhopadhyay, Bin Gao, György Haskó, and Pál Pacher. "Cannabidiol Attenuates Cisplatin-Induced Nephrotoxicity by Decreasing Oxidative/Nitrosative Stress, Inflammation, and Cell Death." *J Pharmacol Exp Ther.* 2009 Mar; 328(3): 708–714.

Chapter 10

1 Grinspoon, Lester MD. *Marihuana Reconsidered*, Bantam Books, May 1971, pg 415.

2 U.S. Statistics Fast Facts. hiv.gov, Minority HIV/AIDS Fund managed by US Department of Health and Human Services, 2019. https://www.hiv.gov/hiv-basics/overview/data-and-trends/statistics, accessed October 3, 2019.

3 Guidelines for the Use of Antiretroviral Agents in Adults and Adolescents Living with HIV. AIDSinfo.nih.gov, US Department of Health and Human Services, 2019. https://aidsinfo.nih.gov/contentfiles/AdultandAdolescentGL003510.pdf, accessed October 3, 2019.

4 Goldberg, Carey. "Brownie Mary' Fights to Legalize Marijuana." *New York Times*, July 6, 1996.

5 Sánchez-Duffhues G1, Calzado MA, de Vinuesa AG, Caballero FJ, Ech-Chahad A, Appendino G, Krohn K, Fiebich BL, Muñoz E. "Denbinobin, a naturally occurring 1,4-phenanthrenequinone, inhibits HIV-1 replication through an NF-kappaB-dependent pathway." *Biochemical Pharmacology*. 2008 Nov 15;76(10):1240-50.

6 de Jong, Bouke C. MD; Prentiss, Diane MA, MPH; McFarland, Willi MD, PhD; Machekano, Rhoderick MPH; Israelski, Dennis M. MD. "Marijuana Use and Its Association With Adherence to Antiretroviral Therapy Among HIV-Infected Persons With Moderate to Severe Nausea." *Journal of Acquired Immune Deficiency Syndrome*, January 1, 2005 Volume 38, Issue 1- pg 43-46.

7 Ethan B. Russo. "Cannabis Therapeutics and the Future of Neurology." *Front Integr Neurosci.* 2018; 12: 51.

8 Fagan SG1, Campbell VA. "The influence of cannabinoids on generic traits of neurodegeneration." *Br J Pharmacol.* 2014 Mar;171(6):1347-60. doi: 10.1111/bph.12492.

9. Xiong W, Cui T, Cheng K, Yang F, Chen SR, Willenbring D, Guan Y, Pan HL, Ren K, Xu Y, Zhang L. "Cannabinoids suppress inflammatory and neuropathic pain by targeting α3 glycine receptors." *Journal of Experimental Medicine.* 2012 Jun 4;209(6):1121-34.

10 Russo, Ethan B. "Cannabis Therapeutics and the Future of Neurology." *Front. Integr. Neurosci.*10 October 2018.

11 Elizabeth A. Penner, MD, MPH, Hannah Buettner, BA, Murray A. Mittleman, MD, DrPHb,. "The Impact of Marijuana Use on Glucose, Insulin, and Insulin Resistance among US Adults." *American Journal of Medicine*, July 2013 Vol. 126 Issue 7, pp. 583-589.

12 McWilliams, Peter. "A Question of Compassion: An AIDS- Cancer Patient Explores Medical Marijuana", Prelude Press, June 1,1998.

Chapter 11

1 Is Marijuana an Effective Treatment for Migraines? David L Bearman MD, in a letter printed in the Feb 3, 2005 edition of Los Angeles City Beat, medicalmarijuana.procon.org, procon.org, 2019. https://medicalmarijuana.procon.org/view.answers.php?questionID=000218, accessed October 3, 2019.

2 Burch RC1, Loder S, Loder E, Smitherman TA. "The prevalence and burden of migraine and severe headache in the United States: updated statistics from government health surveillance studies." *Headache.* 2015 Jan;55(1):21-34.

3 Dickinson, Emily. *The Complete Poems Of Emily Dickinson*, Boston: Little, Brown and Co. 1924 pp.330.

4 Pinja Leimuranta, Leonard Khiroug, and Rashid Giniatullin. "Emerging Role of (Endo)Cannabinoids in Migraine." *Frontiers in Pharmacology*, 2018; 9: 420. Published online 2018 Apr 24.

5 Bryson C. Lochte, Alexander Beletsky, Nebiyou K. Samuel, and Igor Grant. "The Use of Cannabis for Headache Disorders." *Cannabis and Cannabinoid Research.* 2017; 2(1): 61–71.

6 Schiff PhD., Paul L. "Ergot and Its Alkaloids." *Am J Pharm Educ.* 2006 Oct 15; 70(5): 98.

7 Dr. William Brooke O' Shaughnessy. *Bengal Dispensatory and Pharmacopeia (1840).* Calcutta, Bishop's College Press, 1840.

8 Pinja Leimuranta, Leonard Khiroug, and Rashid Giniatullin. "Emerging Role of (Endo)Cannabinoids in Migraine." *Frontiers in Pharmacology*, 2018; 9: 420. Published online 2018 Apr 24.

9 Ethan B. Russo. "Clinical Endocannabinoid Deficiency Reconsidered: Current Research Supports the Theory in Migraine, Fibromyalgia, Irritable Bowel, and Other Treatment-Resistant Syndromes." *Cannabis Cannabinoid Research.* 2016; 1(1): 154–165.

10 Rhyne DN1, Anderson SL1, Gedde M2, Borgelt LM1,3. "Effects of Medical Marijuana on Migraine Headache Frequency in an Adult Population." *Pharmacotherapy.* 2016 May;36(5):505-10.

Chapter 12

1 Gregory T. Carter, MD, Co-director, MDA/ALS Center at the University of Washington Medical Center, Oct. 2003, Muscular Dystrophy Association Biography, medicalmarijuana.procon.org, procon.org, 2019. https://medicalmarijuana.procon.org/view.source.php?sourceID=001437, accessed October 3, 2019.

2 David R. Kumar, BS, Florence Aslinia, MD, Steven H. Yale, MD, and Joseph J. Mazza, MD. "Jean-Martin Charcot: The Father of Neurology." *Clin Med Res.* 2011 Mar; 9(1): 46–49.

3 Multiple sclerosis FAQs: How Many People Have MS?, NationalMSSociety.org, National MS Society, 2019. https://www.nationalmssociety.org/What-is-MS/MS-FAQ-s, accessed October 3, 2019.

4 Daniel M. Hartung, PharmD, MPH, Dennis N. Bourdette, MD, Sharia M. Ahmed, MPH, and Ruth H. Whitham, MD. "The cost of multiple sclerosis drugs in the US and the pharmaceutical industry. Too big to fail?" *Neurology*. 2015 May 26; 84(21): 2185–2192.

5 KP Johnson, BR Brooks, CC Ford, AD Goodman, RP Lisak, LW Myers, AA Pruitt, MA Rizzo, JW Rose, LP Weiner and JS Wolinsky. "Glatiramer acetate (Copaxone): comparison of continuous versus delayed therapy in a six-year organized multiple sclerosis trial." *Multiple Sclerosis* 2003; 9: 585¡/591. www.multiplesclerosisjournal.com.

6 Institute for Clinical and Economic Review (ICER). "Institute for Clinical and Economic Review Releases Evidence Report on Disease-Modifying Therapies for Multiple Sclerosis, including Daclizumab and Ocrelizumab." ICER-review.org, Institute for Clinical and Economic Review, 2019. https://icer-review.org/announcements/ms-evidence-report/, accessed October 3, 2019.

7 Daniel M. Hartung, PharmD, MPH, Dennis N. Bourdette, MD, Sharia M. Ahmed, MPH, and Ruth H. Whitham, MD. "The cost of multiple sclerosis drugs in the US and the pharmaceutical industry. Too big to fail?" *Neurology*. 2015 May 26; 84(21): 2185–2192.

8 I. Wirguin, R. Mechoulam, A. Breuer, E. Schezen, J. Weidenfeld, and T. Brenner. "Suppression of Experimental Autoimmune Encephalomyelitis by Cannabinoids." *Immunopharmacology*, (Nov-Dec 1994), pp. 209-214.

9 Ethan B. Russo. "Clinical Endocannabinoid Deficiency Reconsidered: Current Research Supports the Theory in Migraine, Fibromyalgia, Irritable Bowel, and Other Treatment-Resistant Syndromes." *Cannabis Cannabinoid Research*. 2016; 1(1): 154–165.

10 Novotna, A. ,Mares, J., Ratcliffe, S. , Novakova, I., Vachova, M., Zapletalova, O., Gasperini, C., Pozzillih, C., Cefaro, L., Comii, G., Rossii, P., Amblerk, Z., Stelmasiakl, Z., Erdmannm, A., Montalbann, X., Klimek, A., Davies, P. "Sativex Spasticity Study Group, A randomized, double-blind, placebo-controlled, parallel-group, enriched-design study of nabiximols* (Sativex®), as add-on therapy, in subjects with refractory spasticity caused by multiple sclerosis." *European Journal of Neurology,* 2011Sep;18(9):1122-31.

11 Russo, Ethan B. "Cannabinoids in the management of difficult to treat pain." *Ther Clin Risk Manag.* 2008 Feb; 4(1): 245–259.

Chapter 13

1 Eubanks PhD, Lisa M. "A Molecular Link Between the Active Component of Marijuana and Alzheimer's Disease Pathology." *Molecular Pharmaceutics*, Aug 9, 2006.

2 Alzheimer's Association Facts and Figures (Quick Facts). ALZ.org, Alzheimer's Association®, 2019. https://www.alz.org/alzheimer_s_dementia, accessed October 3, 2019.

3 NIH: national Institute on Aging. Alzheimer's Disease Fact Sheet. NIA.NIH. gov, National Institutes of Health, 2019. https://www.nia.nih.gov/health/alzheimers-disease-fact-sheet, accessed October 3, 2019.

4 Morganti-Kossmann, Maria Cristina PhD; Otto, Viviane I. PhD; Stahel, Philip F. MD; Kossmann, Thomas MD. "The role of inflammation in neurologic disease." *Current Opinion in Critical Care:Neuroscience.* April 2000 - Volume 6 - Issue 2 - p 98-109.

5 Degan D1, Ornello R1, Tiseo C1, Carolei A1, Sacco S1, Pistoia F1. "The Role of Inflammation in Neurological Disorders." *Curr Pharm Des.* 2018;24(14):1485-1501.

6 Russo, Ethan B. "Cannabis Therapeutics and the Future of Neurology." *Frontiers in Integrative Neuroscience.* 2018; 12: 51.

7 Jan Lewerenz1, and Pamela Maher2, "Chronic Glutamate Toxicity in Neurodegenerative Diseases—What is the Evidence?" *Front Neurosci.* 2015; 9: 469.

8 Zi-Qiang Shao. "Comparison of the efficacy of four cholinesterase inhibitors in combination with memantine for the treatment of Alzheimer's disease." *International Journal of Clinical and Experimental Medicine.* 2015; 8(2): 2944–2948.

9 Namenda by Carly Helfand, FiercePharma.com. Questex LLC, 2019. https://www.fiercepharma.com/special-report/namenda, accessed October 3, 2019.

10 Chen H-SV, Lipton SA. "Mechanism of memantine block of NMDA-activated channels in rat retinal ganglion cells: uncompetitive antagonism." *J Physiol (Lond)* 499: 27–46, 1997.

11 Chen HS, Pellegrini JW, Aggarwal SK, Lei SZ, Warach S, Jensen FE et al. "Open-channel block of NMDA responses by memantine: therapeutic advantage against NMDA receptor-mediated neurotoxicity." *J Neurosci* 12: 4427–4436, 1992.

12 Chen HS, Wang YF, Rayudu PV, Edgecomb P, Neill JC, Segal MM et al. "Neuroprotective concentration of the NMDA open-channel blocker memantine are effective without cytoplasmic vacuolization following post-ischemic administration and do not block maze learning or LTP." *Neuroscience* 86: 1121–1132, 1998.

13 Kales H. C., Valenstein M., Kim H. M., McCarthy J. F., Ganoczy D., Cunningham F., et al. . (2007). "Mortality risk in patients with dementia treated with antipsychotics versus other psychiatric medications." *Am. J. Psychiatry* 164, 1568–1576; quiz 1623.

14 Iuvone T., Esposito G., Esposito R., Santamaria R., Di Rosa M., Izzo A. A. (2004). "Neuroprotective effect of cannabidiol, a non-psychoactive component from Cannabis sativa, on β-amyloid-induced toxicity in PC12 cells." *J. Neurochem.* 89, 134–141.

15 Eubanks L. M., Rogers C. J., Beuscher A. E., IV., Koob G. F., Olson A. J., Dickerson T. J., et al. (2006). "A molecular link between the active component of marijuana and Alzheimer's disease pathology." *Mol. Pharm.* 3, 773–777.

16 Azza B. El-Remessy, Ibrahim E. Khalil, Suraporn Matragoon, Gamal Abou-Mohamed, Nai-Jer Tsai, Penny Roon, Ruth B. Caldwell, Robert W. Caldwell, Keith Green, and Gregory I. Liou. "Neuroprotective Effect of(−)Δ9-Tetrahydrocannabinol and Cannabidiol in N-Methyl-d-Aspartate-Induced Retinal Neurotoxicity Involvement of Peroxynitrite." *American Journal of Pathology.* 2003 Nov; 163(5): 1997–2008.

Chapter 14

1 Kassirer MD, Jerome P. "Federal Foolishness and Marijuana." *New England Journal of Medicine*, Jan. 30, 1997.

2 Timothy R. Mhyre, James T. Boyd, Robert W. Hamill, and Kathleen A. Maguire-Zeiss. "Parkinson's Disease." *Subcell Biochem.* 2012; 65: 389–455.

3 Sandeep Vasant More & Dong-Kug Choi. "Promising cannabinoid-based therapies for Parkinson's disease: motor symptoms to neuroprotection." *Molecular Neurodegeneration* volume 10, Article number: 17 (2015).

4 Amantadine, parkinson.org, The Parkinson's Foundation, 2019. https://www.parkinson.org/Understanding-Parkinsons/Treatment/Prescription-Medications/Amantadine-Symmetrel, accessed October 3, 2019.

5 Shabani M, Hosseinmardi N, Haghani M, Shaibani V, Janahmadi M. "Maternal exposure to the CB1 cannabinoid agonist WIN 55212–2 produces robust changes in motor function and intrinsic electrophysiological properties of cerebellar Purkinje neurons in rat offspring." *Neuroscience.* 2011;172:139–52.

6 Venderova K, Ruzicka E, Vorisek V, Visnovsky P. "Survey on cannabis use in Parkinson's disease: subjective improvement of motor symptom." *Movement Disorders.* 2004;19:1102–6.

7 Ex-Cop Larry Smith Treat Parkinson's with Cannabis. youtube.com, Google LLC, 2019. https://www.youtube.com/watch?v=yI1X72RTNLE, accessed October 3, 2019.

8 Kohler, Judith. "More of the legal marijuana sold in Colorado is increasingly for recreational use." *Denver Post*, Aug 6, 2019.

9 Taylor Andrew Finseth, 1 Jessica Louise Hedeman, 1 Robert Preston Brown, II, 2 Kristina I. Johnson, 3 Matthew Sean Binder, 1 and Benzi M. Kluger. "Self-Reported Efficacy of Cannabis and Other Complementary Medicine Modalities by Parkinson's Disease Patients in Colorado." *Evid Based Complement Alternat Med.* 2015; 2015: 874849.

10 REM sleep behavior disorder. MayoClinic.org, Mayo Foundation for Medical Education and Research (MFMER), 2019. https://www.mayoclinic.org/diseases-conditions/rem-sleep-behavior-disorder/symptoms-causes/syc-20352920, accessed October 3, 2019.

11 M. H. N. Chagas, MD PhD, A. L. Eckeli MD PhD, A. W. Zuardi MD PhD, M. A. Pena-Pereira MD, M. A. Sobreira-Neto MD, E. T. Sobreira PhD, M. R. Camilo MD, M. M. Bergamaschi PhD, C. H. Schenck MD, J. E. C. Hallak MD PhD, V. Tumas MD PhD and J. A. S. Crippa MD PhD. "Cannabidiol can improve complex sleep-related behaviors associated with rapid eye movement sleep behavior disorder in Parkinson's disease patients: a case series." *Journal of Clinical Pharmacy and Therapeutics,* Received 25 February 2014, Accepted 23 April 2014.

12 Sinéad Walsh,a Katarzyna Mnich,b Ken Mackie,c Adrienne M. Gorman,b David P. Finn,a and Eilís Dowda. "Loss of cannabinoid CB1 receptor expression in the 6-hydroxydopamine-induced nigrostriatal terminal lesion model of Parkinson's disease in the rat." *Brain Res Bull.* 2010 Apr 5; 81(6): 543–548.

13 Sandeep Vasant More and Dong-Kug Choi, "Promising cannabinoid-based therapies for Parkinson's disease: motor symptoms to neuroprotection." *Molecular Neurodegeneration,* (2015) 10:17 DOI 10.1186/s13024-015-0012-0.

14 Ahlskog PhD MD, Eric J. "Aerobic Exercise: Evidence for a Direct Brain Effect to Slow Parkinson Disease Progression." *Mayo Clinic Proceedings* March 2018 Vol 93, Issue 3, pp 360-372.

Chapter 15

1 Werner, Craig. *Marijuana Gateway to Health. How Cannabis Protects Us from Caner and Alzheimer's Disease.* Dachstar Press, 2011, pp 56.

2 Epilepsy: Key Facts; WHO.int, WHO, 2019. https://www.who.int/news-room/fact-sheets/detail/epilepsy, accessed October 3, 2019.

3. Kirsten M. Fiest, PhD, Khara M. Sauro, PhD, Samuel Wiebe, MD, MSc, Scott B. Patten, MD, PhD, Churl-Su Kwon, MD, Jonathan Dykeman, MD, Tamara Prings-heim, MD, MSc, Diane L. Lorenzetti, PhD, and Nathalie Jetté, MD. "Prevalence and incidence of epilepsy. A systematic review and meta-analysis of international studies." *Neurology.* 2017 Jan 17; 88(3): 296–303.

4 Romigi A, Bari M, Placidi F, et al. "Cerebrospinal fluid levels of the endocan-nabinoid anandamide are reduced in patients with untreated newly diagnosed temporal lobe epilepsy." *Epilepsia.* 2010;51:768–72.

5 Katona I, Freund TF. "Endocannabinoid signaling as a synaptic circuit breaker in neurological disease." *Nat Med.* 2008;14:923–930.

6 Wahab, Abdul. "Difficulties in Treatment and Management of Epilepsy and Challenges in New Drug Development." *Pharmaceuticals* (Basel). 2010 Jul; 3(7): 2090–2110.

7 Geffrey AL1, Pollack SF1, Bruno PL1, Thiele EA1. "Drug-drug interaction be-tween clobazam and cannabidiol in children with refractory epilepsy." *Epilepsia.* 2015 Aug;56(8):1246-51.

8 Tyler E. Gaston E. Martina Bebin Gary R. Cutter Yuliang Liu Jerzy P. Szaflarski for the UAB CBD Program. "Interactions between cannabidiol and commonly used antiepileptic drugs." *Epilepia,* Aug 6 2017.

9 Kerstin Iffland,1 and Franjo Grotenhermen1. "An Update on Safety and Side Effects of Cannabidiol: A Review of Clinical Data and Relevant Animal Studies." *Cannabis Cannabinoid Res.* 2017; 2(1): 139–154.

10 Perucca, Emilio. "Cannabinoids in the Treatment of Epilepsy: Hard Evidence at Last?" *Journal of Epilepsy Research.* 2017 Dec; 7(2): 61–76.

11 Porter BE, Jacobson C. "Report of a parent survey of cannabidiol-enriched cannabis use in pediatric treatment- resistant epilepsy." *Epilepsy & Behavior.* 2013 Dec; 29 (3):574-7.

12 Mazurkiewicz-Beldzinska M, Thiele EA, Benbadis S, et al. "Treatment with cannabidiol (CBD) significantly reduces drop seizure frequency in Lennox-Gastaut syndrome (LGS): results of a multi-centre, rando- mised, double-blind, placebo-controlled trial." (GWPCARE4). 32nd International Epilepsy Congress, 2017 Sep 2 - Sep 6; Barcelona, Spain. *Epilepsia*; In press.

13 Krithiga Sekar. Conceptualization, Writing – Original Draft Preparation1 and Alison Pack, Supervision, Writing – Review & Editinga,1. "Epidiolex as adjunct therapy for treatment of refractory epilepsy: a comprehensive review with a focus on adverse effects." Version 1. *F1000Res.* 2019; 8: F1000 Faculty Rev-234. Published online 2019 Feb 28.

14 Dustin Sulak a, Russell Saneto b, Bonni Goldstein c. "The current status of artisanal cannabis for the treatment of epilepsy in the United States." *Epilepsy and Behavior,* Received 27 September 2016 Revised 16 December 2016 Accepted 17 December 2016.

15 Evan C. Rosenberg,a,1 Pabitra H. Patra,b,1 and Benjamin J. Whalleyb,*. "Therapeutic effects of cannabinoids in animal models of seizures, epilepsy, epileptogenesis, and epilepsy-related neuroprotection." *Epilepsy Behavior.* 2017 May; 70(Pt B): 319–327.

16 Dustin Sulak a, Russell Saneto b, Bonni Goldstein c. "The current status of artisanal cannabis for the treatment of epilepsy in the United States." *Epilepsy and Behavior,* Received 27 September 2016 Revised 16 December 2016 Accepted 17 December 2016.

17 Epidiolex: Highlights of Prescribing Information. www.accessdata.fda.gov, [PDF], https://www.accessdata.fda.gov/drugsatfda_docs/label/2018/210365lbl.pdf, accessed October 3, 2019.

18 Pediatric Cannabinoid Dosing Guidelines [PDF]. theroc.us, Realm of Caring Foundation, Inc. 2019, http://www.theroc.us/images/PediatricGuidelines.pdf, accessed October 3, 2019.

Chapter 16

1 Sagan, Carl. "Carl Sagan as Mr. X" essay written in 1969 for Lester Grinspoon book *Marihuana Reconsidered*, Yale University Press1971, organism.earth, https://www.organism.earth/library/document/9, accessed October 3, 2019

2 Anxiety and Depression of America: Understand the Facts: Facts and Statistics, ADAA.org, Anxiety and Depression Association of America, 2019. https://adaa. org/about-adaa/press-room/facts-statistics, accessed October 3, 2019.

3 Barnhost, Amy. "The Empty Promise of Suicide Prevention." *The New York Times* April 26, 2019, Opinion Page.

4 López-Muñoz F1, Alamo C. "Monoaminergic neurotransmission: the history of the discovery of antidepressants from 1950s until today." *Curr Pharm Des.* 2009;15(14):1563-86.

5 Hillhouse, Todd M., Porter, Joseph H. "A brief history of the development of antidepressant drugs: From monoamines to glutamate." *Experimental Clinical Psychopharmacology.* 2015 Feb; 23(1): 1–21.

6 Daniel Santarsieri and Thomas L Schwartz. "Antidepressant efficacy and side-effect burden: a quick guide for clinicians." *Drugs Context.* 2015; 4: 212290.

7 Depression: How effective are antidepressants? InformedHealth.org, Anxiety and Depression Association of America, 2019.https://adaa.org/about-adaa/press-room/facts-statistics, accessed October 3, 2019.

8 Charles F. Zorumski, Yukitoshi Izumi, and Steven Mennerick, "Ketamine: NMDA Receptors and Beyond." *J Neurosci.* 2016 Nov 2; 36(44): 11158–11164.

9 Sophie Billioti de Gage, PhD student, Yola Moride, professor, Thierry Ducruet, researcher, Tobias Kurth, Hélène Verdoux, professor, Marie Tournier, Antoine Pariente, Bernard Bégaud. "Benzodiazepine use and risk of Alzheimer's disease: case-control study." *British Medical Journal* 2014; 349 (Published 09 September 2014).

10 Alex R. De Mello Schier, Natalai P de Oliveirs Ribeiro,Danielle S. Coutinho, Segio Machado, Oscar Arias-Carrion, Jose A Crippa, Antonie W. Zuardi, Antonie A Nardi and Adriana Silva. "Antidepressant-like and Anxiolytic-Like Effects of Cannabidiol: A Chemical Compound of Cannabis Sativa." *CNS & Neurological Disorders-* Drug Targets, 2014, Vol 13 No 6.

11 Alex R. De Mello Schier, Natalai P de Oliveirs Ribeiro,Danielle S. Coutinho, Se-gio Machado, Oscar Arias-Carrion, Jose A Crippa, Antonie W. Zuardi, Antonie A Nardi and Adriana Silva. "Antidepressant-like and Anxiolytic-Like Effects of Cannabidiol: A Chemical Compound of Cannabis Sativa." *CNS & Neurological Disorders- Drug Targets*, 2014, Vol 13 No 6.

12 Abir T. El-Alfya, Kelly Iveya, Keisha Robinsona, Safwat Ahmedb,1, Mohamed Radwanb, Desmond Sladeb, Ikhlas Khanb,c, Mahmoud ElSohlyb,d, and Samir Rossb,C. "Antidepressant-like effect of Δ9-tetrahydrocannabinol and other can-nabinoids isolated from Cannabis sativa L." *Pharmacol Biochem Behav.* 2010 June ; 95(4): 434–442.

Chapter 17

1 Why I changed my mind on weed by Dr. Sanjay Gupta. CNN.com, Ca-ble News Network, 2019. https://www.cnn.com/2013/08/08/health/gup-ta-changed-mind-marijuana/index.html, accessed October 3, 2019.

2 National Institute of Diabetes and Digestive and Kidney Diseases: Digestive Dis-eases Statistics for the United States. niddk.nih.gov, U.S. Department of Health and Human Services National Institutes of Health, 2019. https://www.niddk.nih.gov/health-information/health-statistics/digestive-diseases, accessed October 3, 2019.

3 Peery AF, Dellon ES, Lund J. "Burden of gastrointestinal disease in the United States: 2012 update." *Gastroenterology.* 2012;143:1179–1187.

4 Nicholas V. DiPatrizio. "Endocannabinoids in the Gut." *Cannabis and Canna-binoid Research.* 2016; 1(1): 67–77. Published online 2016 Feb 1. doi: 10.1089/can.2016.0001.

5 Izzo AA, Coutts AA. "Cannabinoids and the digestive tract." *Handb Exp Pharma-col.* 2005:(168):573-98.

6 Krzysztof Lis, Olga Kuzawińska, and Ewa Bałkowiec-Iskra. "Tumor necrosis factor inhibitors – state of knowledge." *Arch Med Sci.* 2014 Dec 22; 10(6): 1175–1185.

7 Gay Stolberg, Sheryl. "Heartburn Drug Linked to Deaths to be Withdrawn." *The New York Times*, Section A pg15, March 24, 2000.

8 Two New Drugs for Tardive Dyskinesia Hit the Market by Thomas Morrow MD. ManagedCareMag.com, MediMedia, 2019. https://www.managedcaremag.com/archives/2018/1/two-new-drugs-tardive-dyskinesia-hit-market, accessed October 3, 2019.

9 Lim WC, Wang Y, MacDonald JK, Hanauer S. "Aminosalicylates for induction of remission or response in Crohn's disease." (Review), *Cochrane Database of Systematic Reviews*, 2016, Issue 7. Art. No.: CD008870.

10 Florian Bär, Christian Sina, and Klaus Fellermann. "Thiopurines in inflammatory bowel disease revisited." *World J Gastroenterol.* 2013 Mar 21; 19(11): 1699–1706.

11 Ahmed MD, Waseem, Katz MD, Seymour. "Therapeutic Use of Cannabis in Inflammatory Bowel Disease." *Gastroenterol Hepatol* (N Y). 2016 Nov; 12(11): 668–679.

12 Borrelli F, Aviello, G, Romano B, Orlando P, Capsso R, Maiello f, et al. "A safe and non-psychotropic ingrediant of the marijuana plant Cannabis Sativa, is protective in a murine model of colitis." *J. Mol Med* 2009; 87;1111-21.

13 Jamontt JM, Molleman A, Pertwee RG, Parsons ME. "The effects of delta-tetrahydrocannabinol and cannabidiol alone and in combination on damage, inflammation and in vitro disturbances in rat colitis." *British Journal Pharmacol* 2010;60;712-23.

14 Borrelli F, Fasolino I, Romano B,Capasso R, Maireelo F, Coppola D, Orlando P, Battista G, Pagano E, Di Marzo V, Izzo A. "Beneficial effect of the non-psychotropic plant cannabinoid cannabigerol on experimental inflammatory bowel disease." *Biochemical Pharmacology*,85 (2013) 1306-1316.

15 Chesher G, Jackson D. "Anticonvulsant effects of cannabinoids in mice: drug interactions within cannabinoids and cannabinoid interactions with phenytoin." *Psychopharmacology* (Berl) 1974;37:255–264.

16 Karler R, Turkanis SA. "Subacute cannabinoid treatment: anticonvulsant activity and withdrawal excitability in mice." *Br J Pharmacol.* 1980;68:479–484.

Chapter 18

1 Marincolo, Sebastian. *high insights on marijuana*, Dog Ear Press 2010, pg 208.

2 January is Glaucoma Awareness Month. glaucoma.org, Glaucoma Research Foundation, 2019. https://www.glaucoma.org/news/glaucoma-awareness-month.php, accessed October 3, 2019.

3 Glaucoma Facts and Stats. glaucoma.org, Glaucoma Research Foundation, 2019. https://www.glaucoma.org/glaucoma/glaucoma-facts-and-stats.php, accessed October 21, 2019.

4 I Tomida,1 R G Pertwee,2 and A Azuara-Blanco1. "Cannabinoids and glaucoma." *Br J Ophthalmol.* 2004 May; 88(5): 708–713.

5 Hepler RS, Frank IR. Marihuana smoking and intraocular pressure (letter). *JAMA* 1971;217:1392.

6 Drug Update: Vyzulta and Rhopressa, aao.org, American Academy of Ophthalmology, 2019. https://www.aao.org/eyenet/article/drug-update-vyzulta-and-rhopressa, accessed October 3, 2019.

7 Joshua D. Stein, MD, MS,1 Nakul Shekhawat, MD, MPH,1 Nidhi Talwar, MA,1 and Rajesh Balkrishnan, PhD.2. "Impact of the Introduction of Generic Latanoprost on Glaucoma Medication Adherence." *Ophthalmology.* Author manuscript; available in PMC 2016 Apr 1.

8 Noecker, Robert. "The management of glaucoma and intraocular hypertension: current approaches and recent advances." *Ther Clin Risk Manag.* 2006 Jun; 2(2): 193–206.

9 Scherer WJ. "A retrospective review of non-responders to latanoprost." *J Ocul Pharmacol Ther.* 2002;18:287–91.

10 Lester Grinspoon, M.D. and James B. Bakalar. *Marijuana The Forbidden Medicine*, Yale University Press 1997, pg 49.

11 Zielinski, Graema. "Activist Robert C. Randall Dies." *Washington Post* June 8, 2001. Sourced WashingtonPost.com, https://www.washingtonpost.com/archive/local/2001/06/08/activist-robert-c-randall-dies/c6e832a4-55e2-47fc-a3c8-5e011da66e04/, accessed October 3, 2019.

12 Straiker A, Maguire C, Makie K, et al. "Localization of cannabinoid CB1 receptors in the human anterior eye and retina." *Invest Ophthalmol Visual Sci* 1999;40:2442–8.

13 Huestis, Marilyn A. "Human Cannabinoid Pharmacokinetics." *Chem Biodivers.* 2007 Aug; 4(8): 1770–1804.

Chapter 19

1 Gorton Carruth and Eugene Ehrlich. *American Quotations*, Wing Books, 1992 pg 269.

2 Beat Lutz,1 Giovanni Marsicano,2,3 Rafael Maldonado,4 and Cecilia J. Hillard5. "The endocannabinoid system in guarding against fear, anxiety and stress." *Nat Rev Neurosci*. 2015 Dec; 16(12): 705–718.

3 Tringale MD, Rolando, Jensen MD, Claudia. "Cannabis and Insomnia." *O'Shaughnessy's* Autumn 2011 pg 31.

4 Feinberg I, Jones R, Walker J, Cavness C, Floyd T. " Effects of marijuana extract and tetrahydrocannabinol on electroencephalographic sleep patterns." *Clin Pharmacol Ther*. 1976 Jun;19(6):782-94.

5 Thropy, Michael J. "Classification of Sleep Disorders." *Neurotherapeutics*. 2012 Oct; 9(4): 687–701.

6 Love, Dr. Richa (@drrichalove). Original post: "One of my patients is 36-yr male veteran who says CBD oil has done wonders for his sleep. He now gets a full night's rest and is less often disturbed by nightmares. Check out this link to learn more about medical cannabis for sleep https://zurl.co/jtwg. #insomnia #sleep #mmj" conversation with Colleen Higgins (@ColleenHiggy) 12:32 PM - 22 May 2019, https://twitter.com/drrichalove/status/1131281711923322880, accessed October 27, 2019.

7 The 'Sleepy' Cannabinoid CBN Might Not Actually Be Sedating by Meg Hartley. leafly.com, Leafly, 2019. https://www.leafly.com/news/health/is-cbn-cannabinoid-sedating, accessed October 3, 2019.

8 Signs and Symptoms of Untreated Lyme Disease. CDC.gov, Centers for Disease Control and Prevention, 2019. https://www.cdc.gov/lyme/signs_symptoms/index.html, accessed October 3, 2019.

9 Xiong W1, Cui T, Cheng K, Yang F, Chen SR, Willenbring D, Guan Y, Pan HL, Ren K, Xu Y, Zhang L. "Cannabinoids suppress inflammatory and neuropathic pain by targeting α3 glycine receptors." *Journal of Experimental Medicine*. 2012 Jun 4;209(6):1121-34.

10 Azza B. El-Remessy, Ibrahim E. Khalil, Suraporn Matragoon, Gamal Abou-Mohamed, Nai-Jer Tsai, Penny Roon, Ruth B. Caldwell, Robert W. Caldwell, Keith
Green, and Gregory I. Liou. "Neuroprotective Effect of(−)Δ9-Tetrahydrocannab-
inol and Cannabidiol in N-Methyl-d-Aspartate-Induced Retinal Neurotoxicity
Involvement of Peroxynitrite." *American Journal of Pathology*. 2003 Nov; 163(5):
1997–2008.

11 Statistics About Diabetes Overall Numbers, diabetes.org, American Diabetes Association, 2019. https://www.diabetes.org/resources/statistics/statistics-about-di-
abetes, accessed October 3, 2019.

12 Insulin Costs. C-Span.org, National Cable Satellite Corporation, 2019. Originally aired April 10, 219 2:49:00. https://www.c-span.org/video/?459672-1/insu-
lin-costs, accessed October 3, 2019.

13 G Gruden, F Barutta, G Kunos,and P Pacher. "Role of the endocannabinoid system in diabetes and diabetic complications." *Br J Pharmacol*. 2016 Apr; 173(7):
1116–1127.

14 F. J. Bermúdez-Silva & J. Suárez & E. Baixeras & N. Cobo & D. Bautista & A.
L. Cuesta-Muñoz & E. Fuentes & P. Juan-Pico & M. J. Castro & G. Milman &
R. Mechoulam & A. Nadal & F. Rodríguez de Fonseca. "Presence of function-
al cannabinoid receptors in human endocrine pancreas." *Diabetologia* (2008)
51:476–487.

15 Pacher P, Beckman JS, Liaudet L. "Nitric oxide and peroxynitrite in health and
disease." *Physiol Rev* 2007, 87:315–424.

16 Béla Horváth, Partha Mukhopadhyay, György Haskó, and Pál Pacher. "The
Endocannabinoid System and Plant-Derived Cannabinoids in Diabetes and
Diabetic Complications." *The American Journal of Pathology*, Vol. 180, No. 2,
February 2012.

17 Khalid A. Jadoon1, Stuart H. Ratcliffe2, David A. Barrett3, E. Louise Thomas4,
Colin Stott5, Jimmy D. Bell4, Saoirse E. O'Sullivan1 and Garry D. Tan. "Emerging Technologies and Therapeutics. Efficacy and Safety of Cannabidiol and Tet-
rahydrocannabivarin on Glycemic and Lipid Parameters in Patients With Type
2 Diabetes: A Randomized, Double-Blind, Placebo-Controlled, Parallel Group
Pilot Study." *Diabetes Care* 2016 Oct; 39(10): 1777-1786.

18 Sarfaraz S, Afaq F, Adhami VM, Mukhtar H. "Cannabinoid receptor as a novel
target for the treatment of prostate cancer." *Cancer Res*. 2005;65:1635–41.

19 Juan A. Ramos and Fernando J. Bianco1. "The role of cannabinoids in prostate cancer: Basic science perspective and potential clinical applications." *Indian J Urol.* 2012 Jan-Mar; 28(1): 9–14.

20 Sami Sarfaraz, Farrukh Afaq, Vaqar M. Adhami, and Hasan Mukhtar. "Cannabinoid Receptor as a Novel Target for the Treatment of Prostate Cancer." *Department of Dermatology*, University of Wisconsin, Madison, Wisconsin.

Chapter 20

1 Gorton Carruth and Eugene Ehrlich. *American Quotations,* Wing Books, 1992 pg 377.

2 Dr. Jack E. Henningfield of the National Institute of Drug Abuse (NIDA) and Dr. Neal L. Benowitz of the University of California at San Francisco (UCSF), data from an article in the *New York Times* (August 2, 1994, p. C3).

3 Xinqi Zhoua, Kaeli Zimmermannb, Fei Xina, Weihua Zhaoa, Roelinka T. Derckxb, Anja Sassmannshausenb, Dirk Scheeleb, Rene Hurlemannb, Bernd Weberc,d, Keith M. Kendricka, Benjamin Beckera, "Cue Reactivity in the Ventral Striatum Characterizes Heavy Cannabis Use, Whereas Reactivity in the Dorsal Striatum Mediates Dependent Use." *Biological Psychiatry: Cognitive Neuroscience and Neuroimaging*, August 2019, Vol 4, Issue 8, pg 751-762.

4 J. Eric Fleming, MD and Sean Lockwood, MD. "Cannabinoid Hyperemesis Syndrome." *Fed Pract.* 2017 Oct; 34(10): 33–36.

5 twitter.com. Dr.Michael Verbora (@mverbora), Tweeted 6:58AM-24 Jul 2019 from Toronto, Ontario.

6 Monte AA1, Shelton SK2, Mills E2, Saben J2, Hopkinson A2, Sonn B2, Devivo M2, Chang T2, Fox J2, Brevik C2, Williamson K2, Abbott D2. "Acute Illness Associated With Cannabis Use, by Route of Exposure: An Observational Study." *Ann Intern Med.* 2019 Mar 26.

7 Cecilia J. Sorensen,1 Kristen DeSanto,2 Laura Borgelt,3 Kristina T. Phillips,4 and Andrew A. Monte1,5,6, "Cannabinoid Hyperemesis Syndrome: Diagnosis, Pathophysiology, and Treatment—a Systematic Review." *J Med Toxicol.* 2017 Mar; 13(1): 71–87.

Conclusion

1 Bob Marley: Lifestyle (Life of the Legend). bobmarley.com, Bob Marley, 2013. http://www.bobmarley.com/history/, accessed October 3, 2019.

2 Senators held a hearing to remind you that 'good people don't smoke marijuana' (yes, really) by Christopher Ingraham, Washington post.com, The Washington Post, 2019. https://www.washingtonpost.com/news/wonk/wp/2016/04/05/sena-tors-one-sided-marijuana-hearing-is-heavy-on-anecdote-light-on-data, accessed October 3, 2019.

3 NBCNews.com. Health News, Linda Carroll and Lauren Dunn, $2.1 million drug to treat rare genetic disease approved by FDA by Linda Carroll and Lauren Dunn. NBCNews.com. NBC Universal, 2019. https://www.nbcnews.com/health/health-news/2-1-million-drug-treat-rare-genetic-disease-approved-fda-n1009956, accessed October 3, 2019.

4 Schmader, Davis, *Weed, The User's Guide A 21st Century Handbook for Enjoying Marijuana*. Sasquatch Books, April 2016.

Index

Made in the USA
Las Vegas, NV
07 November 2022

58983280R00184